D1614921

Principles of
Toxicological Pathology

Principles of Toxicological Pathology

John R. Glaister

Hazleton Laboratories (Europe) Ltd.,
Harrogate, England

Taylor & Francis
London and Philadelphia
1986

UK	Taylor & Francis Ltd, 4 John St., London WC1N 2ET
USA	Taylor & Francis Inc., 242 Cherry St., Philadelphia, PA 19106-1906

British Library Cataloguing in Publication Data

Glaister, John R.
    Principles of toxicological pathology.
    1. Toxicology — Technique
    I. Title
    615.9′0028   RA1211

ISBN 0-85066-316-4

Library of Congress Cataloging in Publication Data is available

Typeset by Electronic Village Ltd, Richmond, Surrey
Printed in Great Britain by
Redwood Burn Limited, Trowbridge, Wiltshire

Contents

Acknowledgements

This book was possible only because of the efforts and publications of hundreds of toxicologists and pathologists during the toxicology boom of the last 20 years. The book is largely a reflection of their diligence in making toxicology the scientific discipline that it is today, and hopefully will encourage other scientists in this exciting field. I would also like to thank members of the Hazleton staff for their encouragement, the many pathologists in various institutions for their review and comment on the draft manuscript and the editorial staff of Taylor & Francis for the final polishing. Special thanks are due to Judith Walwyn for literature retrieval, to Sue Morgan for typing the first draft and numerous revisions, and to Margaret Manning for the illustrations. Finally, my wife Cathy and daughter Vicki deserve special mention for their support, and for enduring periods of recluse, frustration and bad temper.

Preface

This book is not intended to be a comprehensive academic treatise. It is an attempt to improve communication and understanding between people interested or involved in toxicology, particularly in regulatory toxicology. For undergraduate students, there is a global view across the principles of toxicological pathology and their application in two main areas of interest, target organ pathology and the pathology of laboratory animals. This should provide the framework for answers to examination questions, but details will have to be gleaned from references listed in the bibliography. For practising toxicologists, the aim is to give them an understanding of the complex language frequently used by their pathologist colleagues. Hopefully they will no longer be overwhelmed by terms such as acute suppurative inflammation or distal axonopathy. In return a pathologist may expect toxicologists to be more understanding and sympathetic in areas of diagnostic uncertainty and not always to insist on reducing the dynamic processes in pathology to fixed numbers for statistical evaluation. Practising pathologists looking for an encyclopaedia will be disappointed. For them, it is an opportunity to sit back from the minutiae of a rare exotic tumour and reconsider the principles and concepts to which they are working. This can be a sobering process, and will hopefully lead to a better understanding of the needs of the toxicologist whom they ultimately serve. Finally, the author would urge the readers to communicate with him if the book displays areas of error, ignorance, misunderstanding or glaring omissions.

John Glaister
Harrogate, May 1985

1. Methods in pathology

Pathology is the science of disease. It is the study of the causes of cell and tissue injury and the ways in which cells and tissues respond to injury. The cause and effect of injury is the basic theme of this book. There are many causes of cell and tissue injury, including biological agents such as viruses and bacteria and physical causes such as extreme heat or cold. Toxicology is concerned predominantly with one class of causal agents, chemicals, and their effect on living systems. The reaction to injury is usually seen as changes in cell or tissue function or as changes in structure. Chemically induced structural changes are the main effect of interest in toxicological pathology, but before these are described in detail the basic tools that the pathologist uses to detect effects will be outlined and their application in toxicology discussed.

Detecting effects

Most organisms are composed of cells, and cells consist mainly of molecules organised into complex subcellular systems. Structural effects caused by chemicals may occur at any level of this biological organisation, literally from molecule to mammal. Three basic techniques are used to detect structural effects at these different levels: electron microscopy (EM), light microscopy (LM) and post mortem (PM) (Figure 1.1).

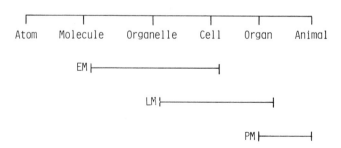

Figure 1.1. Operating ranges of the three basic techniques in pathology.

1

The theoretical resolving power of the electron microscope is about 0.2 nm, which is close to atomic dimensions. In practice, the instrument usually operates between 10 nm and 100 μm (0.1 mm) which is in the range from large molecules to whole cells. Light microscopy covers the range from 1 μm to 10 mm. This is the range from the larger subcellular organelles such as mitochondria to whole cross-sections of some of the smaller organs. Finally, the unaided eye can detect structural changes exceeding 1 mm. This together with the weighing of organs is the principle means of observation in post mortems in which whole organs are examined. Alternative names commonly used for post mortem are autopsy and necropsy.

Most of the emphasis in this book will be on light microscopy and necropsy as basic techniques for detecting effects in toxicological pathology because these are the ones most commonly used. Light microscopy, or histopathology as it is often known, is particularly important since it covers much of the middle of the range from molecule to mammal. Many of the diagnoses used in pathology are based on the light-microscopic examination of tissue sections stained with two dyes, haematoxylin and eosin. Haematoxylin is a basic dye and stains acidic molecules such as DNA blue. This blue staining is known as basophilia. Conversely, the acidic dye eosin stains basic materials, notably proteins, red or pink; and this is known as eosinophilia or acidophilia. These two stains (HE) enable the histopathologist to identify different cell structures and also the shape, size and organisation of the different cells that make up the structure of whole organs. They also enable the histopathologist to detect deviations from normal cell structure and organisation resulting from chemical injury. Detailed accounts of the technical aspects of these methods are listed in the bibliography.

Predicting effects

The toxic effects of most concern are those affecting man and his environment. Direct study of these effects is often difficult, and it is preferable to try to predict the potential adverse effects of chemicals before they are released for use. Most toxicological work therefore uses experimental models, and the results are extrapolated to predict the possible effect of chemicals in man or other target species of interest.

The utility of pathology to detect toxic effects in predictive modelling depends on the type of model used. Models fall into two classes, specific models and general models. Specific models are used to assess a single defined response, for instance organophosphate inhibition of acetylcholinesterase, or the Ames test for detecting mutations in Salmonella. Many specific models use *in vitro* techniques, and biochemical or pharmacological responses are common endpoints in these assays. Pathology plays little or no role in many of these specific models unless structural changes such as kidney damage are of specific interest.

However, a new chemical substance could have one of several hundred possible effects and it would require a huge battery of specific models to screen for this potential toxicity. This is clearly uneconomical and general models play a major role in the assessment of toxicity of new chemicals. The question being addressed in the use of general models is, 'does the chemical at some dose level have any toxic potential that may pose a risk to man or other species?'. In other words, the general model has to detect possible biochemical, functional or morphological responses in any organ of the body. This is clearly an impossible ideal, but the combined use of necropsy and light micoscopy on tissues from laboratory animals is unrivalled in its ability to detect a wide range of responses for predictive toxicology. Some of the reasons for this include:

(1) The use of laboratory animals is an *in vivo* model. The pharmacokinetic (dose) and pharmacodynamic (response) components of this model are thus more likely to be predictive of those in man than many of the possible *in vitro* general models such as tissue culture.

(2) The *range of organs* examined. Virtually every organ in an animal's body can be weighed *post mortem* and examined by naked eye and by light microscopy at reasonable cost. The range of biochemical and pharmacological assays that can be conveniently applied tends to be restricted to a few organs. Similarly, within any one organ a diverse range of structural changes such as cell growth or cell death can be detected by a single assay procedure. A battery of biochemical or pharmacological assays may be needed to sample the range of possible functional responses to injury.

(3) The *resolution* of the assay. Using the combined techniques of necropsy and light microscopy the structure of each organ may be examined from the gross level down to the level of the larger subcellular organelles. This covers much of the scale of potential structural damage from molecule to mammal at reasonable cost.

(4) The *sensitivity* of the assay is often comparable with that of biochemical and pharmacological studies of the same organ. For example, the dose producing liver-cell damage detectable by elevations of serum transaminases is often similar to that causing structural damage detectable by light microscopy. Organ weights are also a sensitive assay. An increase in liver weight, for example, is a good indicator of adaptive change associated with the metabolism and elimination of chemicals.

The application of pathology assays, together with certain biochemical and functional studies in laboratory animals, is currently the most powerful tool available for screening new chemicals for toxic effects. The continued development of *in vitro* methods is a desirable goal, but they are unlikely to replace laboratory animals as general models in the foreseeable future. The value of assays in animals is reflected in various government regulations which require animal safety tests on new chemical substances such as drugs, pesticides and industrial chemicals before they can be used or sold. Compliance with such regulations is often called regulatory toxicology. This is the largest branch of toxicology and the area from which the principles, and some of the problems, of toxicological pathology will be illustrated. Chapter 3 is devoted to structural changes seen in organs that are often targets of toxicity and Chapter 4 reviews common patterns of background pathology in some of the frequently used species. Chapter 5 briefly summarises certain statistical techniques used to evaluate pathology data. First of all, however, some of the basic principles of general pathology that apply to all these chapters have to be described. These, the causal mechanisms and responses to injury, form the basis of Chapter 2.

Bibliography

Bancroft, J. D. (ed.) (1982) *Theory and Practice of Histological Techniques*. (Edinburgh: Churchill Livingstone)

Bancroft, J. D. and Cook, H. C. (1984) *Manual of Histological Techniques*. (Edinburgh: Churchill Livingstone)

Barr, W. T. and Williams, E. D. (1983) Technical and quality assurance in histopathology. *Med. Lab. Sci.*, 40: 257.

Collan, Y. and Romppanen, T. (eds.) (1982) *Morphometry in Morphological Diagnosis*. (Kuopio: Kuopio University Press)

Ghadially, F. N. (1982) *Ultrastructural Pathology of the Cell and Matrix*. (Woburn: Butterworths)

Golberg, L. (ed.) (1983) *Structure–Activity Correlation as a Predictive Tool in Toxicology: Fundamentals, Methods and Applications*. (New York: Hemisphere)

Grice, H. C. (1972) The changing role of pathology in modern safety evaluation. *CRC Crit. Rev. Toxicol.*, 1: 119.

Heywood, R. (1983) Target organ toxicity II. *Toxicol. Letts.*, 18: 83.

Kluwe, W. M. (1981) Renal function tests as indicators of kidney injury in subacute toxicity studies. *Toxicol. Appl. Pharmacol.*, 57: 414.

Macri, A. and Silano, V. (1982) Toxicological and ecotoxicological premarketing testings of chemicals intended for different uses. In *Animals in Toxicological Research*, edited by I. Bartosek, A. Guaitani and E. Pacei (New York: Raven Press)

Mehlman, M., Cramner, M. F. and Shapiro, R. E. (eds.) (1977) Proceedings of the Conference on the Status of Predictive Tools for Application to Safety Evaluation, Present and Future (Carcinogenesis, Mutagenesis). *J. Environ. Pathol. Toxicol.*, 1/2: 1.

Miller, F. J., Graham, J. A. and Gardner, D. E. (1983) The changing role of animal toxicology in support of regulatory decisions. *Environ. Health Perspect.*, 52: 169.

Mitruka, B. M., Rawnsley, H. M. and Vadehra, D. (1976) *Animals for Medical Research: Models for the Study of Human Disease*. (New York: Wiley)

Plaa, G. L. and Hewitt, W. R. (1982) Detection and evaluation of chemically induced liver injury. In *Principles and Methods of Toxicology*, edited by W. A. Hayes (New York: Raven Press)

Purchase, I. F. H. (1982) ICPEMC. working paper 2/6: An appraisal of predictive tests for carcinogenicity. *Mutat. Res.*, 99: 53.

Rees, K. R. (1980) Cells in culture in toxicity testing: a review. *J. Roy. Soc. Med.*, 73: 261.

Reichsman, F. P. and Calabrese, E. J. (1978) Animal extrapolation in environmental health: its theoretical basis and practical applications. *Rev. Environ. Health*, 3: 59.

Reuber, M. D. (1977) Necropsy of animals for scientific research. *Clin. Toxicol.*, 10: 111.

Rowe, V. K., Wolf, M.A., Weil, C.S. and Smyth, H. F. (1959) The toxicological basis of threshold limit values. 2. pathological and biochemical criteria. *Am. Ind. Hyg. Assoc. J.*, 20: 346.

Ward, J. M. and Reznik, G. (1983) Refinements of rodent pathology, and the pathologists' contribution to evaluation of carcinogenesis bioassays. *Prog. Exp. Tumor Res.*, 26: 266.

Wheater, P., Burkitt, G., Daniels, V. and Deakin, P. (1979) *Functional Histology.* (Edinburgh: Churchill Livingstone)

Zapp, J. A. (1977) Extrapolation of animal studies to the human situation. *J. Toxicol. Environ. Health*, 2: 1425

Zbinden, G. (1980) Predictive value of pre-clinical drug safety evaluation. In *Clinical Pharmacology and Therapeutics, Proceedings of the First World Conference on Clinical Pharmacology and Therapeutics*, (New York: Macmillan)

Zbinden, G. (1981) Scope and limitations of animal models for the prediction of human toxicity. In *Organ-directed Toxicity*, edited by S. S. Brown and D. S. Davies (Oxford: Pergamon Press)

2. General pathology

Despite the apparent complexity of toxicological pathology, the principles are simple. Chemicals can produce injury by effects on the cell or on the environment of the cell, and there are three basic histopathological responses to injury. This theme is expanded in this chapter and its practical application in the fields of target-organ pathology and laboratory-animal pathology forms the basis of Chapters 3 and 4.

Mechanism of injury	Response to injury
Intracellular	Degeneration
Extracellular	Proliferation
	Inflammation/repair

The biochemical mechanisms leading to injury at the molecular level are diverse and complex. In principle, they fall into two main categories: injury initiated by the chemical acting on the target cell, and injury that is primarily the result of extracellular mechanisms. These intracellular and extracellular processes are sometimes described as direct or primary and indirect or secondary mechanisms of toxicity. This concept of intracellular and extracellular mechanisms is convenient, but it should be appreciated that a chemical may injure cells by more than one mechanism depending on the nature and extent of exposure and the character of the target organism or tissue.

The cellular events following injury at the molecular level are as diverse as those leading up to it. Our understanding of these early events is sparse and we can only describe with any certainty some of the later and grosser sequelae that can be observed with the electron and light microscope. At this level it is an old axiom in pathology that the number of ways in which cells and tissues can respond to injury is limited. There are two main categories. The first is the response in the injured cells, that is the intracellular response. The second category of response is an extracellular reaction to the presence of the injured cells.

Intracellular responses fall into two main groups. They may be regressive changes such as a decrease in cell size or in the number of organelles. These processes are grouped into the general category known as degeneration. Conversely, cellular components or the cells themselves may increase in size and number as a sequel to injury at the molecular level. Such responses are grouped into the category of proliferations. Finally, the body may react to the presence of abnormal or dying cells by attempting to remove or repair the damage. These extracellular processes are categorised under the general heading of inflammation. This triad of '-ations' — degeneration, proliferation and inflammation — is the foundation upon which a large part of the description of effects in toxicological pathology is built and upon which much of this book is based.

Intracellular mechanisms of injury (Figure 2.1)

Chemical cytotoxicity is most frequently caused by a chemical or a derivative acting directly on the cell and interfering with critical molecular functions. If the molecular malfunction persists, it will ultimately manifest as a biochemical, functional or morphological alteration in the cell. For most toxic chemicals we know very little about the interactions occurring at the molecular level or the mechanisms by which these interactions subsequently lead to the deleterious effects detectable as toxicity. However, to illustrate some of the many potential mechanisms the following are a few brief examples of some of the ways in which chemicals or their reactive metabolites may lead to cell dysfunction. A more detailed exposition of the biochemical mechanisms of toxicity is given by Timbrell (1982).

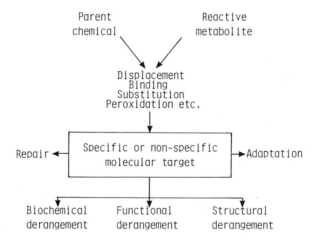

Figure 2.1. Intracellular mechanisms of injury.

Parent chemical

Chemicals may react with the molecular components of cells either specifically or non-specifically and through reversible or irreversible reactions. They may react with the cell membrane, at specific intracellular sites or randomly (Figure 2.2). There are four intracellular systems thought to be particularly critical to a cell's survival. The osmotic and fluid homeostasis of the cell and its organelles are dependent on the integrity of cell membranes. The integrity of the DNA is important for the function of the cell and also for the normal functioning of daughter cells following cell division. Proteins are important both as enzymes and as structural components, and finally, virtually all cellular activity is dependent on an adequate level of energy production.

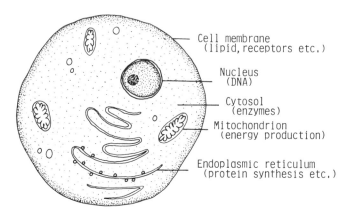

Figure 2.2. Common target sites for chemical injury.

Membranes

Membranes are a critical feature of cell organisation, structure and function. They separate intracellular compartments and separate the cell from the extracellular environment. They also provide the framework upon which enzymes and other proteins function. Effects on membranes feature strongly in many types of chemical toxicity. Direct effects on membranes may be non-specific such as alterations of lipid–protein or lipid–lipid relationships or specific effects on receptors and transport sites.

Volatile general anaesthetics act non-specifically and reversibly on cell membranes. The precise mechanism by which they cause anaesthesia is unknown. There is a positive correlation between anaesthetic potency and oil/water partition coefficient, the ability to reduce surface tension, and the ability to stabilise water clathrates, all of which relate to the physical factors that determine hydrophobicity. Detergents also act non-specifically on lipid membranes. They interfere with ionic bonding of the lipoprotein membrane and so alter the conformation and permeability of the cell. They can also affect membrane-bound organelles and dissociate nucleoprotein complexes in organelles such as ribosomes. The effect of detergents on membranes thus ranges from a reversible dissociation to irreversible destruction depending on the nature and concentration of the detergent.

In contrast, many chemicals have specific effects on membrane lipids, proteins and receptors. This is the basis of many toxicities, particularly neurotoxicity. For example, botulinus toxin binds to peripheral cholinergic presynaptic axon terminals and blocks the release of acetylcholine. Cobra neurotoxin binds to the postsynaptic receptors of neuromuscular junctions rendering them insensitive to acetylcholine.

DNA

Chemicals can affect the structure and function of DNA in several ways. They may bind to it or interfere with the pathways leading to DNA synthesis. The antibiotic actinomycin D is a potent teratogen. It blocks DNA transcription by intercalating between base pairs of DNA via specific hydrogen bonding with the 2-amino group of guanine. Acridine dyes such as proflavin are also intercalating agents. They are planar molecules of similar dimensions to those of normal base pairs and by spreading and distorting the helix cause addition or deletion of bases during DNA replication (frameshift mutation).

Chemicals may covalently bind to DNA, for example the alkylating agents ethanemethanesulphonate and the nitrogen mustards. These compounds are mutagenic largely via alkylation of position 7 of guanine. Chemicals may covalently link various components of DNA. This cross-binding can take basically three forms: down a single helix strand, between the two helix strands and between one helix strand and a protein. Such linkages may seriously compromise the structure and function of DNA.

In addition to hydrogen bonding and covalent bonding, chemicals may interfere with the fidelity of DNA by becoming incorporated into the strand during synthesis and replication. The thymine analogue, 5-bromouracil is the classic example. 5-bromouracil has to be converted metabolically to the deoxyribose triphosphate derivative before incorporation and this illustrates the important point that a chemical may progress through one or more steps before exerting a critical effect. Thus the distinction between the effects of parent chemicals and active metabolites is not always clear cut. DNA synthesis or fidelity can also be modified by chemicals acting on the supply of components for DNA assembly. For example, the dihydrofolate reductase inhibitor methotrexate prevents the availability of single carbon fragments required for thymine synthesis and another analogue of uracil, 5-fluorouracil, inhibits the enzyme thymidine synthetase, thus blocking the synthesis of thymine. In these cases, the effect on DNA is a consequence of chemical activity elsewhere in the cell and this type of effect is sometimes referred to as indirect toxicity. This usage of terminology should not be confused with the use of indirect toxicity for cell injury due to extracellular mechanisms.

Proteins

Chemicals may interfere with the synthesis or functions of proteins. Protein synthesis is a complex multistep process, any stage of which is a potential target for chemical intervention. Cycloxheximide, streptomycin and lincomycin interfere with synthesis at the level of RNA translation. Cycloheximide interferes with the transfer of tRNA to ribosomes and lincomycin inhibits the attachment of tRNA to the ribosome. Streptomycin binds with and causes misreading of mRNA.

Substrate or co-factor depletion or antagonism can also depress protein synthesis. Ethionine is a hepatotoxic analogue of the amino acid methionine. Methionine in the form of S-adenosyl methionine acts as a methyl donor, a process that includes the recycling of adenine. When S-adenosyl ethionine is formed, the recycling is reduced and the subsequent shortage of adenine leads to ATP depletion followed by inhibition of protein synthesis. One effect is to depress the production of the apolipoprotein complex required for hepatic triglyceride secretion. Accumulation of triglycerides in the liver cell cytoplasm eventually leads to fatty liver.

The effect of chemicals on specific proteins or enzymes can have diverse effects. For example, tubulin is an important structural protein involved in cell division, contraction, movement and other processes such as phagocytosis. All of these can be blocked by vinca alkaloids acting on tubulin.

Energy production

Like DNA and protein synthesis, this is also a complex multistage process, with many potential targets for disruption. Chemicals may inhibit or uncouple oxidative phosphorylation or inhibit or deplete the supply of co-factors required for ATP synthesis. Fluoroacetate for example blocks the tricarboxylic acid (TCA) cycle through a process termed lethal synthesis. Fluoroacetate first requires metabolism to fluoroacetyl CoA. This is incorporated into the TCA cycle in an analogous manner to acetyl CoA combining with oxaloacetate to produce fluorocitrate. Fluorocitrate cannot be dehydrated by aconitase, and the TCA cycle is blocked at this point. Cyanide disrupts cell respiration by blocking the electron transport process. It combines with the ferric iron atom in haem proteins destroying their capacity to undergo oxidation and reduction during electron transfer and thereby blocks oxidative phosphorylation and respiration.

Reactive metabolites

Whilst many chemicals have the inherent ability to react with cellular macromolecules, other chemicals require biotransformation to produce a more reactive molecule. In some cases the reactive metabolite is always produced and cell injury is predictable and dose dependent. In other cases, one particular species or genotype may metabolise the chemical by an unusual route or at an abnormal rate and in these cases injury is usually unpredictable. The two major classes of reactive metabolite are electrophilic compounds and free radicals. These may bind covalently to critical macromolecules at various target sites or alternatively initiate destructive processes such as lipid peroxidation (Figure 2.3).

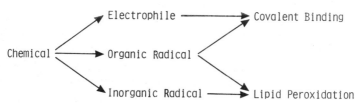

Figure 2.3. Proposed mechanisms of injury by reactive metabolites.

Electrophiles

Electrophilic metabolites are frequent causes of cell and tissue injury by covalent binding to critical macromolecules such as proteins, nucleic acids and small molecular weight substances like ATP. Many of the biotransformation reactions are oxygenations, catalysed by the microsomal mixed function oxidases (MFO). Reactions may involve metabolic attack at various points in the parent chemical such as on carbon, nitrogen or sulphur atoms. The epoxidation of benzpyrene and other cyclic aromatic hydrocarbons is one example of the oxidation of carbon to generate arylating species capable of reacting with DNA to produce mutations. Similarly, aflatoxin B_1, a potent naturally occurring hepatocarcinogen, is thought to be activated by epoxidation of the distal furan ring (Figure 2.4).

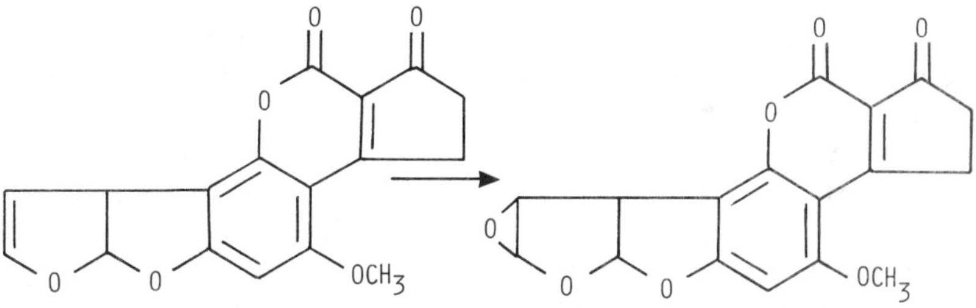

Figure 2.4. Epoxidation of aflatoxin B_1.

Many aromatic amines and amides are carcinogenic following N-oxidation. N-hydroxylation of acetylaminofluorene is one well-studied example. N-hydroxylation is also an important metabolic route for non-carcinogenic toxins such as the hepatotoxins paracetamol and isoniazid, and the methaemoglobin-inducers derived from aniline and other aromatic amines. Metabolic attack on sulphur is less frequently encountered. Oxidative desulphuration of carbon disulphide to release a reactive form of sulphur probably plays an important role in the hepatotoxicity of this compound and similar reactions occur during metabolism of the insecticide Parathion.

Free radicals

A free radical is a molecule or atom with an unpaired electron in its outer shell.

They may be organic or inorganic. Formation of free radicals may be via addition or loss of an electron or by homolytic cleavage of a covalent bond. One-electron reduction of many chemicals to yield free radicals is catalysed by microsomal NADPH-cytochrome C (P-450) reductase. The free radical itself may initiate damage, but under aerobic conditions the radical may react with molecular oxygen to regenerate the parent compound and release the superoxide anion (O_2^-). Superoxide is relatively stable and unlikely to be the main toxic species. Derivatives such as hydrogen peroxide (H_2O_2) and the hydroxyl radical $(OH\cdot)$ are more reactive. $OH\cdot$ is highly reactive and may damage many critical molecules. The redox cycling and generation of active oxygen species is the mechanism by which paraquat is thought to damage the lung (Figure 2.5). Quinone-containing compounds, such as the cardiotoxic antibiotic adriamycin, also readily undergo redox cycling in biological systems, producing O_2^- as a consequence.

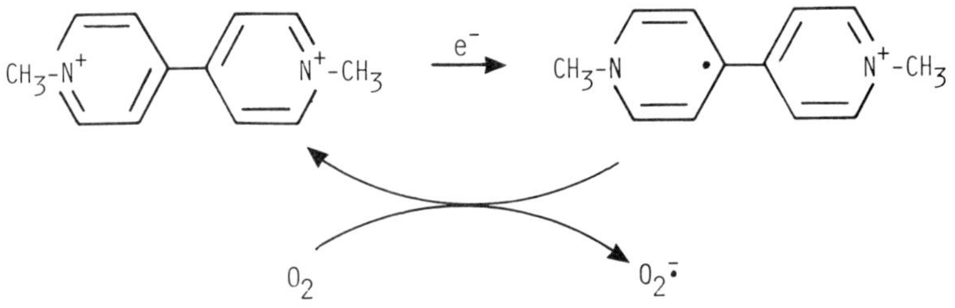

Figure 2.5. Paraquat redox cycling.

If the active oxygen species are not removed by vitamin E and other free-radical scavengers or by enzymes systems such as superoxide dismutase they may initiate cytotoxic processes including lipid peroxidation. Peroxidation of unsaturated lipids is a chain reaction which proceeds in three stages — initiation, propagation and termination (Figure 2.6). The final breakdown products of peroxidation are various lipid alcohols and aldehydes, and some very short-chain products such as malonaldehyde. Some of these products are toxic and may serve to spread the injury to cell sites remote from the site of initiation. The effects of lipid peroxidation are diverse. They include damage to lipid membranes, cross linking between lipids and protein and destruction of enzyme activity by the interaction of their sulphydryl groups with the products of lipid peroxidation.

Whilst generation of active oxygen species is one consequence of free radical generation, the organic radical itself may initiate lipid peroxidation or alternatively covalently combine with macromolecules to exert a deleterious effect. For example CCl_4 is transformed to the trichloromethyl radical $CCl_3\cdot$ through reductive dehalogenation by cytochrome P-450. This would be expected to bind covalently to neighbouring molecules, either to N- or S- atoms or across double bonds and may be an important contributor to cell injury. In short, biotransformation of xenobiotics to free radicals may have several consequences for the cell, both locally at the site of radical production as a result of covalent binding and lipid

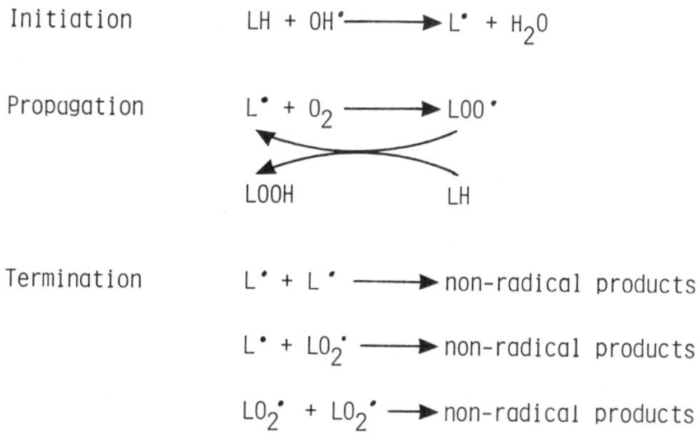

Initiation $\qquad LH + OH^\bullet \longrightarrow L^\bullet + H_2O$

Propagation $\qquad L^\bullet + O_2 \longrightarrow LOO^\bullet$

$\qquad\qquad\qquad$ LOOH $\qquad\qquad$ LH

Termination $\qquad L^\bullet + L^\bullet \longrightarrow$ non-radical products

$\qquad\qquad\qquad L^\bullet + LO_2^\bullet \longrightarrow$ non-radical products

$\qquad\qquad\qquad LO_2^\bullet + LO_2^\bullet \longrightarrow$ non-radical products

Figure 2.6 Stages in lipid peroxidation. LH = Polyunsaturated lipid; L· = Lipid radical

peroxidation, and at other sites due to the diffusion of toxic products of lipid peroxidation.

Finally, free radicals can also be generated by γ, UV and X-irradiation, and are important elements in cutaneous toxicology. Certain halogenated salicylanilides once used as topical bacteriostats are known to cause skin injury. Some of these compounds produce free radicals after ultraviolet irradiation and these may be responsible for initiating injurious lipid peroxidation (phototoxicity) or alternatively form a covalent complex with skin proteins and incite an allergic reaction (photoallergy).

Extracellular mechanisms of injury

All cells are dependent on many factors in their extracellular environment for survival. Chemicals may modify these external factors and thereby produce changes in cell structure or function. Cell injury caused by such chemicals is thus a consequence of extracellular mechanisms and is often referred to as indirect or, secondary injury. In some cases, these secondary effects are relatively minor in comparison with the primary extracellular effect. In other cases, the secondary effects are dominant and appear as target organ toxicity. There are two broad, overlapping groups of extracellular factors related to cell survival and function, those associated with the basic metabolic needs of the cell and those concerned with regulation of cell activity. The former include oxygen and nutrients and the latter hormones and other regulatory substances.

Metabolic mechanisms

The basic metabolic requirements for cell survival are a need for oxygen for energy production and a need for nutrients for both energy production and cell growth. The cells also need an optimal extracellular fluid environment with respect to electrolyte and acid–base composition to support intracellular energy-generating processes and other critical functions especially at the cell membrane. The extracellular fluid is also important as a means of removing waste products produced during energy generation and other metabolic processes. Oxygen and nutrient supply, fluid and electrolyte balance, and waste product removal are critical to all cells, and the body's needs are supported by special organ systems upon which all cells are dependent (Figure 2.7).

These major organ systems supporting metabolism at the cellular level, and cellular metabolism and function itself are interdependent. They in turn are regulated by various other systems, notably neural and endocrine. This illustrates the overlap and considerable complexity that may be found when studying extracellular mechanisms of cellular injury. An in-depth knowledge of normal physiology is an essential prerequisite to unravelling the complexity of some of the relationships between cause and effect. Inevitably, much of this complexity in pathophysiology has to be ignored when illustrating the basic principles, but it should not be forgotten. As a final introductory point, it should be noted that in some cases, chemical injury may result in generalised effects on many cells and tissues in the body and in others it may appear organ-specific if the cells of that organ are critically dependent on specific extracellular factors.

Oxygen

Oxygen deprivation is a very common cause of cell and tissue injury. Adequate oxygen supply to the cell depends on adequate ventilatory function, adequate diffusion from alveoli into blood, adequate numbers of functional erythrocytes and an adequate cardiovascular system to transport oxygenated erythrocytes to the cell. Any one or more of these sites may be the target site for chemical attack. For example, airway obstruction may be caused by the inhalation of severe irritants such as toluene diisocyanate, and diffusion of oxygen from alveolar air into blood may be reduced by paraquat and other chemicals which damage the alveolar lining cells. A reduction in the number of functional erythrocytes may result from lack of erythrocyte production in bone marrow damaged by chemicals or from interference with the oxygen-carrying capacity of the erythrocyte. Examples of the latter are production of carboxyhaemoglobin by carbon monoxide and methaemoglobin by nitrites. All these examples result in a primary oxygen deficiency in the circulating blood and this condition is known as hypoxia. All cells in the body are at risk to this type of oxygen deprivation, but the cells most at risk are those with high oxygen requirements such as the brain, heart, liver and kidney. As these are critical life support systems, death of the whole organism will follow severe oxygen deprivation (anoxia). If the oxygen deprivation is not severe and life threatening, the organism will compensate through various mechanisms such as increased heart and respiration rate. These and other compensatory mechanisms may be adequate to maintain body function, but in other cases compensation may be inadequate and result in slow progressive damage

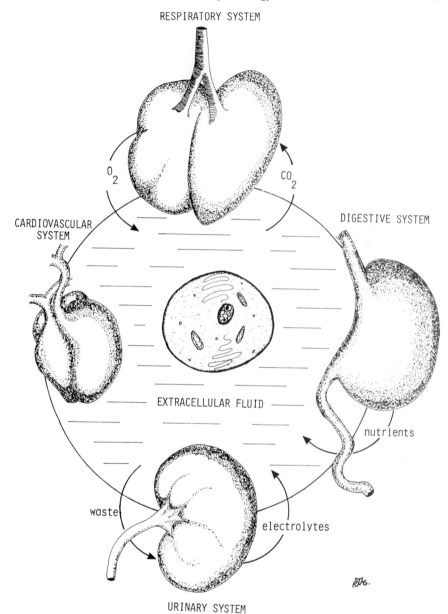

RESPIRATORY SYSTEM

O_2 CO_2

CARDIOVASCULAR SYSTEM

DIGESTIVE SYSTEM

EXTRACELLULAR FLUID

nutrients

waste

electrolytes

URINARY SYSTEM

Figure 2.7 Major organ systems supporting metabolic requirements at the cellular level.

to vital organs such as the liver.

A second type of anoxia is ischaemic anoxia. In this type, the blood is adequately oxygenated, but blood flow to cells is reduced. Blood flow reduction may be generalised throughout the body or localised to specific tissues. Cardiac arrest from toxic substances is an obvious cause of inadequate generalised blood flow, and extreme hypotension following administration of vasodilating chemicals has similar effects. In both cases the heart and brain are at risk and subtained blood flow reduction leads to death of the whole organism, often so rapidly that there is little or no discernible structural damage to the cells. In contrast, in localised disruption of blood flow the organism often survives and damage becomes obvious in the affected organ. For example, obstruction of blood vessels by intravenous injection of large particles or air bubbles may lead to death of tissue supplied by the obstructed vessel. Materials that physically block blood vessels are often referred to as emboli, e.g. fat emboli, air emboli and tumour emboli. Obstruction of blood vessels may also result from coagulation of blood itself, a process known as thrombosis. In toxicology, this is most frequently seen after intravascular injection of irritant chemicals. In rodents, the end of the tail may die and drop off if an irritant is injected into tail vessels causing thrombosis and reduction of blood flow to the tip of the tail. Thrombosis may also occur as a more subtle side effect of chemicals such as after the long term administration of high-oestrogen contraceptive pills. In conclusion, there are many ways in which oxygen supply can be reduced by toxic chemicals and these can lead to death of cells, tissues and whole organisms depending on the nature, rate and extent of the oxygen deprivation.

Nutrients

Nutrients are used by all cells for metabolic reactions to provide energy or building blocks for cell growth and cell function. Like the supply of oxygen to the cell, the supply of nutrients is a multistep process. It comprises ingestion, digestion, absorption and finally transport of absorbed nutrients to the cell membrane. Chemicals may interfere with one or more of these processes depriving cells of essential nutrients and potentially leading to cell injury. The type of effect observed depends on the nature, rate and extent of nutrient deficiency and ranges from a generalised effect on the whole organism to effects on specific cell types.

The most common effect in toxicity studies is a generalised one, usually related to interference with ingestion. Some chemicals administered in diet are unpalatable. The animals refuse to eat their food and lose weight. A similar effect may occur following administration of chemicals acting on the central nervous system. A drowsy, ataxic or paralysed animal may not eat. This generalised effect is obvious as a decrease in body weight or as a failure to gain weight at the normal rate. The response at the cell and tissue level is a similar reduction in size or growth with the main exception of the testes. These maintain spermatogenesis and the testis to body weight ratio usually increases in fasting animals. Apart from these anomalies in organ weights, the main problem facing the pathologist is accumulation of fat in the liver cells as a result of fat mobilisation from adipose depots. This is usually minor, but may mimic fat accumulation produced by toxins acting directly on fat metabolism in the liver cells. To the clinical chemist, the main problem is an increase in blood urea nitrogen due to excessive protein catabolism. This may mimic the effect of renal toxins. Other causes of generalised nutrient deficiency are vomiting and diarrhoea which interfere with digestion and absorption. This often occurs in dogs and primates, but rats do not vomit.

In contrast to generalised nutrient deprivation, some chemicals may interfere with the supply of specific nutrients. As cell requirements frequently vary from organ to organ damage may occur preferentially in specific organs. Deficiency of vitamins, trace elements and essential amino acids and fatty acids are the most commonly encountered effects of chemicals. For example, anticonvulsant drugs may leads to malabsorption of folic acid. If continued, folic acid deficiency eventually leads to abnormal red cell production in bone marrow and ultimately to megaloblastic anaemia. Similarly, prolonged oral administration of fatty or oily materials may interfere with the absorption of fat soluble vitamins and precipitate deficiency syndromes if the dietary concentrations of vitamins are marginal.

An equally serious problem in toxicology is excess nutrients, particularly in long-term rodent studies. Rodents are usually allowed unrestricted access to diets that are frequently rich in protein. This leads to overnutrition. Overnutrition enhances some of the important diseases of ageing rodents such as renal disease and tumours. Reducing the protein level in the diet will reduce the degree of renal disease in ageing animals. Restriction of the amount of daily diet available often has a similar effect and reduces the frequency of certain tumour types. The relationship between nutrition and disease is also being extensively investigated in man, with interesting results such as the correlation between high fat diets and some of the common human cancers.

Other effects

Fluid and electrolyte balance and elimination of the waste products of cellular metabolism are potential targets for chemicals, but these processes are complex and the effects on the animal are likely to be generalised such as fluid retention (oedema) or dehydration. However, more specific effects may occur, for example, in man following laxative abuse. This may lead to secondary structural changes in the kidney due to chronic depletion of sodium, potassium and body water.

Regulatory mechanisms

The activity of cells needs to be regulated and integrated to satisfy the requirements of the organism as a whole. There are several interrelated regulatory systems in the body, any of which may be the target for chemicals. The nervous, endocrine and immune systems are the ones most frequently affected by chemicals.

Nervous system

This is the most critical of all the regulatory systems, directly or indirectly affecting all cells in the body. Widespread acute disruption or damage to this system has diverse effects and if excessive will be lethal. In other cases, the effect in the nervous system may be more subtle, and secondary changes may develop in organs innervated by specific parts of the nervous system. The main effects likely to be seen are those related to neural control of muscle contraction or of glandular secretion.

Certain classes of pesticides and other chemicals can damage peripheral nerves such as the sciatic nerve in the leg. The muscle supplied by this nerve is no longer stimulated to contract and it withers away. This process is known as atrophy. Since one nerve fibre innervates many muscle fibres it may be easier to detect the muscle change than the damaged nerve fibres, and the affect may mimic primary muscle disease. Other chemicals affect the autonomic system and may change the rate and extent of glandular secretion. Many people have experienced the dry mouth caused by reduced salivary secretion following atropine premedication. This is a short-term effect, but long-term reduction of lachrymal secretion by anticholinergics will lead to a dry eye, and ultimately permanent eye damage. Similarly, persistent cholinergic stimulation of gastric acid secretion may damage the lining of the stomach.

Endocrine system

This is the second major regulatory system in the body. The system regulates general factors common to all cells such as growth and fluid and electrolyte balance. It also has specific regulatory control over other organ systems like the reproductive system. Chemically-induced generalised effects are uncommon, but effects on specific organs are sometimes encountered in toxicity studies. Testicular function, for example, is regulated mainly by the gonadotrophins LH and FSH secreted by the pituitary gland. Non-steroidal compounds such as methallibur suppress gonadotrophin secretion causing inhibition of spermatogenesis and atrophy of the accessory sex glands. These secondary changes in the reproductive tract are striking in comparison with the subtle morphological effects in the pituitary. Hormone assays may be required to distinguish between primary and secondary chemical toxicity in cases such as these.

Even more difficult to unravel is the effect of long-term low grade endocrine imbalance that may lead to an increased incidence of tumours in endocrine-dependent tissues. This problem is particularly prevalent in long-term toxicity studies in the rat which are one of the main bioassays for potential carcinogens. Much of the spontaneous background pathology of ageing rats is associated with endocrine-related tissues. Increased incidences of tumours in endocrine organs or in dependent tissues such as the mammary gland are fairly common outcomes in these studies. Since these studies are part of the regulatory decision-making process, such results provoke considerable debate about whether the chemical is acting as a genotoxic carcinogen by interacting with DNA or whether it is a non-genotoxic carcinogen operating by epigenetic mechanisms such as chronic endocrine imbalance. This debate continues and as yet there is no universal satisfactory solution. It does, however, indicate the importance of understanding the significant role that indirect or secondary mechanisms can play in toxicological pathology.

Immune system

The immune system regulates foreign molecules entering the body and foreign molecules generated within the body. Not all molecules are recognised as foreign by the immune system but if they are, they are termed antigens. Commonly encountered antigenic molecules are associated with bacteria, viruses, foreign proteins and chemicals. In the normal course of events these antigens are neutralised by the immune system and eliminated without causing any adverse effect on the host. Under other circumstances, the immune response is excessive and detrimental to the host. This detrimental response ranges from a local effect such as a rash to a severe fatal generalised reaction. These detrimental immune reactions are referred to as hypersensitivity or allergic reactions. They are an important mechanism in chemical toxicity.

The classification of allergic reactions as extracellular or secondary is equivocal since low molecular weight chemicals are rarely antigenic unless attached to cell or tissue components. However, the major component of cell injury affects extracellular systems and it is convenient to consider immune-mediated injury as an indirect effect. Allergic reactions are conventionally divided into four classes, three classes primarily comprising circulating antibodies produced by cells of the immune system and the fourth mediated by attack on foreign molecules by cells themselves. Chemicals may evoke any one of these four classes of allergic reactions.

In Type I reactions, initial exposure incites IgE antibody production. IgE localises on the surface of mast cells. A second exposure to the antigenic chemical causes release of vasoactive substances after the antigen combines with the antibody on the surface of the mast cell. The extent of the mast cell release reaction depends on the nature of exposure to the chemical. It may be localised causing local swelling, or generalised causing bronchial constriction, vomiting, diarrhoea, acute collapse and possibly death. The acute generalised reaction is known as anaphylactic shock. There are considerable interspecies differences in the manifestation of anaphylaxis. Bronchial smooth muscle is the target organ in guinea-pigs, whereas the target organs in the dog are the liver and gut. Penicillin is the prototype chemical causing Type I reactions in man.

In Type II reactions, the antigen rather than the antibody is associated with the cell surface. Subsequent antibody production and complexing with surface-bound antigen leads either to direct destruction of the cell through activation of the complement system or to attack by phagocytic cells which recognise surface-bound antibodies. This type of allergy is also known as the cytotoxic type. It is classically associated with destruction or removal of circulating blood cells leading to anaemia or thrombocytopenia. Penicillin is again the prototype example of this type of reaction for the red cell, and quinidine is the classic sensitiser of platelets.

Antibody-antigen reactions also form the basis of Type III allergy. In contrast to Types I and II, this does not include the cell surface in the initial stages. The antibody reacts with antigen in the blood or extracellular fluid to form immune complexes. Under certain conditions, the complexes deposit on or around cells leading to cell damage. In this case, the cells and tissues are 'innocent bystanders' and injury is truly the result of indirect mechanisms. In some cases the immune complexes aggregate in the walls of blood vessels such as those in the renal glomeruli and the joints producing a generalised reaction known as serum sickness. Drugs that may produce serum sickness include sulphonamides, penicillins, phenylbutazone and streptomycin. In other cases the complexes may deposit on circulating blood cells leading to haemolytic anaemia and other effects similar to those produced by Type II reactions.

Type IV allergic reactions are mediated by direct cellular attack on foreign molecules. The movement of cells into tissues and their effects are slower than those of antibodies and reactions mediated by cells are often referred to as delayed hypersensitivity. These reactions are an important aspect of cutaneous toxicology. Many chemicals will complex with components of the skin, causing the components to be recognised by the immune system as foreign molecules. Subsequent exposure to these chemicals produces immune-cell infiltration and release of tissue-damaging agents leading to dermatitis (eczema) if the exposure is persistent. Nickel, formaldehyde and many other simple chemicals are examples of potent skin sensitisers.

The above classification is useful to illustrate the principles of immune injury (Figure 2.8), but it must be emphasised that allergic reactions in man are often less well defined, particularly when investigating target organ injury such as hepatotoxicity or nephrotoxicity. In many cases there may be evidence of an immune reaction such as increased circulating eosinophils, or antibodies directed against the target organ, but the relative role of these as mediators of injury rather than as side-effects of direct cytotoxic injury is often difficult to unravel. This brings us back to one of the central themes of the book. It is important to understand causal mechanisms of injury, but for specific chemicals these are often unknown and much of toxicological pathology is related to the description of effects and then speculating about mechanisms. The next sections are devoted to descriptions of the main cell and tissue responses to injury; namely, degeneration, proliferation, inflammation and repair.

Degeneration

Degenerations are one of the three ways in which cells and tissues may respond to injury. Degenerations are regressive changes within a cell or population of cells. They include a diverse spectrum of morphological responses ranging from adaptive homeostasis to irreversible changes such as cell death. Numerous bizarre structural changes may be seen by electron microscopy but, using the conventional

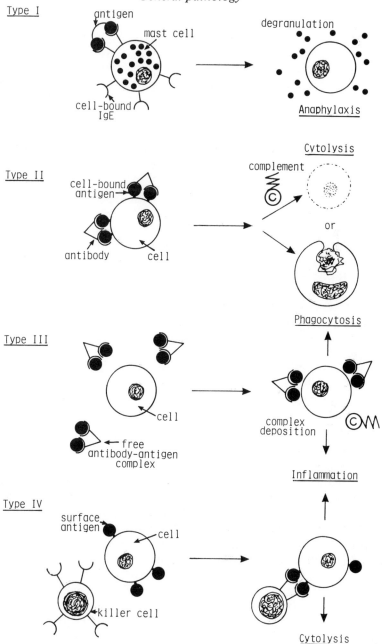

Figure 2.8 Mechanisms of immune injury.

light microscope, the most common regressive changes are reduced cell size or growth (atrophy), intracellular accumulations and cell death (necrosis).

Atrophy

This is a simple decrease in cell size or number, usually causing a shrinkage of affected tissues and organs. Atrophy implies some adverse environment requiring the cell to regress to a smaller size, at which level it survives, but usually at a lower level of function. Secondary mechanisms of cellular injury, such as reduced blood supply, denervation and nutrient or endocrine deficiency are the main causes of this adverse environment and subsequent cell shrinkage. In many cases, atrophy is an adaptive homeostatic response to the adverse environment and is reversible provided the cause is eliminated or deficiencies restored. However, the most common single type of atrophy is atrophy of old age, and this ageing process is not reversible.

At the ultrastructural level, the decrease in cell mass is seen as a breakdown of cell components. These components are digested intracellularly by a process known as autophagocytosis. Autophagocytosis is often incomplete, particularly when the cell is trying to degrade cell membranes, and intracellular residual bodies remain. These ultimately appear by light microscopy as brown pigment known as lipofuscin. If this pigmentation is extensive, it may be visible at necropsy as a brown discoloration of the whole organ, termed 'brown atrophy'.

Intracellular accumulations

An essential component of cell function or survival is the ability to maintain equilibria between intracellular compartments and between the cell and its external environment. Chemicals and other injurious agents may disturb these equilibria and materials may accumulate in the cytoplasm or organelles of the cell. The most commonly encountered intracellular accumulations are water, fat and various types of inclusions (Figure 2.9).

Water

Cellular swelling due to influx of sodium and water into the cell is a common reversible morphologic response to a variety of forms of injury. It may also be the early stage of processes leading ultimately to cell death. The intracellular sodium concentration in mammalian cells is much lower than in the extracellular fluid. This differential is maintained by an ATP energy-dependent 'sodium pump' within the cell membrane. This pump also maintains intracellular potassium at a higher level than in the extracellular fluid. The pump can be inhibited specifically or non-specifically. For example, ouabain inhibits the membrane enzyme ATPase used in this active transport system. Hypoxia or mitochondrial poisons disrupt energy cycles, depleting ATP and non-specifically inhibit the membrane sodium pump. With hypoxia, there is an initial rapid loss of potassium from the cell followed by a gradual increase in intracellular sodium and calcium and a decrease in magnesium. Accompanying the sodium influx is an iso-osmotic gain of intracellular water causing swelling of the cell.

When all cells of an organ are affected the organ usually appears pale and the

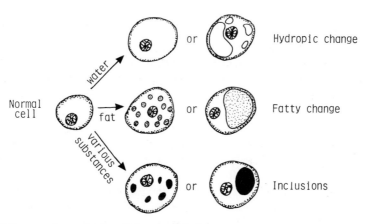

Figure 2.9 Common types of intracellular accumulations.

overall weight is increased. Histologically, the mild forms of cellular swellings are difficult to distinguish, but ultrastructurally the endoplasmic reticulum is dilated and mitochondria may be swollen. Severe cellular swelling produces small clear vacuoles or single large vacuoles in the cytoplasm known as hydropic change. In extreme cases, vacuoles may burst leading to death of the cell. Such severe hydropic changes are most common in the parenchymal organs with high metabolic activity such as kidney, liver and heart. Examples include hydropic vacuolation of the proximal convoluted tubules of the kidney in hypokalemia and liver cell vacuolation in carbon tetrachloride poisoning. Accumulation of water also occurs after death. It is often difficult to distinguish post-mortem autolytic or agonal changes from true ante-mortem effects, especially at the ultrastructural level.

Fat

Fatty change is the accumulation of fat in non-fatty tissues, notably those with a high metabolic rate such as liver. It is sometimes referred to as steatosis and although frequently reversible, it may forebode cell death. The increase in intracellular lipid implies an imbalance in the production, mobilisation or utilisation of lipid within the affected cell. Chemicals may affect any one or more of these components of lipid metabolism via intracellular or extracellular mechanisms. Since fatty change in the liver is such a frequent response to chemicals, these mechanisms are considered in more detail in Chapter 3.

A minor degree of fatty change is not discernible at necropsy except perhaps as an increase in organ weight. In severe cases the affected organs appear yellow and feel greasy. Histologically, the fatty change appears as sharply demarcated empty vacuoles of various sizes. The vacuoles are empty because the intracellular fat dissolves in the solvents used in processing tissues to paraffin sections. Demonstration of actual fat droplets requires the preparation of frozen sections to avoid the use of solvents and then staining the sections with fat-soluble stains such as Oil red O or Sudan IV. It is important to recognise that fat accumulates normally in some cells, for example in the sinusoidal (Ito) cells of monkey liver, in bile duct epithelial cells in the dog and in the kidney tubules of the cat. These normal variants should not be mistaken for pathological fatty change.

Inclusions

Intracellular accumulations of granular or solid materials are known as inclusions. This is a broad term encompassing pigments, hyaline droplets and other materials. Pigments are self-coloured materials in the cytoplasm which are visible without staining. They are fairly common in toxicity studies in laboratory animals and usually appear brownish in the sections. Their origin and nature are diverse and the precise identification of these pigments is a specialised and often difficult process. The inclusions most frequently associated with chemical toxicity are haemosiderin and bilirubin, derived from breakdown of haemoglobin, and lipofuscin and myelinoid bodies derived from intracellular membranes.

Haemosiderin is a golden-yellow to brown, granular or crystalline, iron-containing pigment. The iron can be demonstrated using stains such as Perl's Prussian Blue. Recycling of iron from the breakdown of effete circulating red cells is a normal physiological process, and the spleen and liver in several species normally contain stainable iron. However, excessive red cell breakdown leads to storage of excess iron as haemosiderin. Excessive red cell breakdown may be local as in areas of haemorrhage or widespread due to chemicals attacking circulating red cells and causing anaemia. Haemosiderin accumulation is not a true degeneration, but a secondary effect of red cell destruction. It generally does not impair cell or organ function.

Bilirubin is the iron-free breakdown product of the haem component of haemoglobin and is normally excreted as a yellow-green-brown pigment in bile. The amount of bilirubin can increase by increasing red cell destruction, by damaging the liver cells that excrete it, or by blocking the bile ducts along which it is conducted to the intestine. The excess bilirubin may be visible clinically or at necropsy as a yellow discoloration of various tissues termed jaundice. In severe conditions excess bilirubin may precipitate in liver cells and associated intercellular channels and appear histologically as green-brown to black globular deposits.

Lipofuscin is the pigment most commonly associated with membrane degradation. It was mentioned in association with atrophy, but it may also occur following other forms of persistent injury such as cirrhosis of the liver. Current evidence suggests that lipofuscin is the end product of free-radical peroxidation of polyunsaturated membrane lipids. The presence of lipofuscin in cells of animals in toxicity studies usually suggests low-grade persistent chronic injury.

Myelinoid bodies are another type of cytoplasmic inclusion derived from membrane phospholipids. Ultrastructurally, myelinoid bodies are lysosomes containing phospholipids arranged either as densely packed concentric lamellae, reticular formations or crystalloid structures. Histologically, they may appear as granules or impart a foamy appearance to the cytoplasm as in phospholipidosis caused by cationic amphiphilic drugs.

Aggregates of protein are another type of inclusion likely to be observed with light microscopy. Proteins have many basic groups and therefore an affinity for eosin. Aggregates appear as bright eosinophilic granules or droplets in the cytoplasm. The homogeneous, glassy deposits are often referred to as hyaline droplets. The causes are numerous. For example, droplets of reabsorbed protein may occur in renal proximal tubular cells if excess protein leaks through the glomeruli. In chronic alcoholism in man the hepatocytes may develop cytoplasmic droplets referred to as alcoholic hyaline.

Necrosis

Necrosis means death of cells while still forming part of the living body and it is a very common response to chemical injury. It is the end result of a variety of mechanisms, both intracellular, such as lethal synthesis, and extracellular such as hypoxia. It is one of the most significant life-threatening sequels to chemical injury and the intracellular events associated with cell death have been extensively investigated by biochemists, electron microscopists and histopathologists. Histologically, necrosis is characterised by a sequence of morphological changes which, in contrast to biochemical and ultrastructural changes, take several hours to develop after the actual death of the cell. Two processes are associated with these morphological changes: enzymic lysis of the cell and denaturation of protein. If denaturation of protein is the most prominent process, the basic outline of the cell and tissue is preserved for a considerable time and the necrosis is termed coagulative. If lysis predominates, the tissue become softened and the necrosis is called liquefactive or colliquitive. Coagulative necrosis is common in most tissues, but liquefactive necrosis occurs in the brain, occasionally at other sites and in association with a form of inflammation known as suppuration.

Biochemical changes

Biochemists have had many problems in defining the critical molecular events following lethal injury. A host of biochemical changes such as inhibition of oxidative phosphorylation, protein synthesis, the function of ion pumps and of many other cell functions can be found following injury known to cause cell death. Unfortunately, inhibition of many cell functions can be achieved to a similar degree by other chemicals and the cell will survive, thus casting doubt on the critical nature of these events. Despite these difficulties, there are two major classes of agent that lead to acute cell death followed by necrosis: agents that inhibit or uncouple oxidative phosphorylation; and agents that disrupt the permeability and transport mechanisms of the cell membrane. Current investigations suggest that a critical event linking many of the biochemical and morphological changes ultimately leading to cell death is a rapid increase in cytosolic calcium. No matter what type of lethal injury the cell undergoes, calcium accumulation occurs, resulting either from impaired energy metabolism or from plasma membrane alterations. Calcium is an extremely important regulator of diverse intracellular activities and any excessive flux in ionised calcium levels will exert a deleterious effect on the cell and initiate catabolic processes leading to cell death. Whether calcium influx turns out to be the final common pathway in all injuries leading to cell death is, however, still to be determined.

Ultrastructural changes

Electron microscopists have been investigating the earlier events in necrosis to try to define and understand the critical structural pertubations leading to death of the cell. Numerous ultrastructural changes have been described shortly after lethal cell injury. For example, early ultrastructural changes caused by hypoxic injury include disappearance of mitochondrial calcium granules, the formation of blebs along the cell membrane, depletion of cytoplasmic glycogen and clumping of nuclear chromatin. Other changes include shrinkage and then swelling of mitochrondria and dilation and disruption of endoplasmic reticulum. These ultimately progress to the complete degradation of cell components visible by light microscopy. This progression of ultrastructural changes following hypoxic injury has been divided into several stages, the first few of which are reversible. The stage in which the mitochondria begin to show high-amplitude swelling is considered the 'point of no return', beyond which the cell will not survive. In contrast to hypoxic injury, toxic injury by carbon tetrachloride is seen initially in the smooth endoplasmic reticulum (SER). The primary change is swelling due to influx of water and this is soon followed by degranulation of the rough endoplasmic reticulum (RER). Mitochondrial and other organelle damage occurs subsequently to the changes in the endoplasmic reticulum. These data suggest that the rate and sequence of progression of ultrastructural changes associated with the early stages of cell death may vary according to cell type and to the type of injury and that it will be impossible to define a single common pathway of events.

Histological changes

In coagulative necrosis, changes are seen in both the nucleus and cytoplasm. Nuclear changes are the hallmark of cell death and usually occur in one of two basic patterns, karyolysis and pyknosis. In karyolysis, the nucleus gradually fades and dissolves leaving a ghost outline. This change probably reflects activation of RNAases and DNAases as the pH of the cell drops. Pyknosis is characterised by nuclear shrinkage and increased staining intensity. Subsequently the nucleus may fragment to form small basophilic granules. This process is termed karyor-rhexis. In the cytoplasm, oxidative respiration ceases and there is a build-up of lactic acid and a fall in pH. The breakdown of structural components of the cytoplasm releases further acidic groups and consequently the cytoplasm stains intensely acidophilic (Figure 2.10). Ultimately, most necrotic cells and cell debris disappear, by a combined process of enzymic digestion and phagocytosis by white blood cells. In some circumstances, the necrotic cells tend to attract calcium salts and other minerals which precipitate on the dead cell. This process is known as dystrophic mineralisation and appears histologically as basophilic granules or globules in HE stained sections.

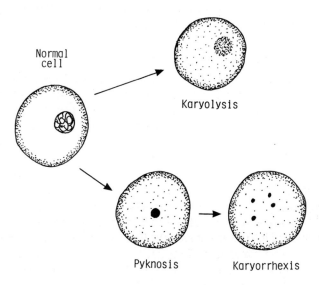

Figure 2.10. Histological stages in coagulative necrosis.

Other terms associated with necrosis are single cell necrosis, necrobiosis, piece-meal necrosis, caseous necrosis and infarct. Single cell necrosis, as the name implies, is characterised by isolated necrotic cells. The term necrobiosis describes a necrotic process that appears to occur in a gradual manner and affects a single or a few cells. Piecemeal necrosis is a term sometimes used for necrobiosis in the liver in which isolated necrotic cells are associated with a few mononuclear cells. Caseous necrosis is a distinctive form of coagulative necrosis classically associated with tuberculous infection. The necrotic tissue appears white, granular and cheesy at autopsy — hence the term caseous. An infarct is a zone or area of necrosis caused by disruption of the arterial blood supply such as thrombosis of a branch of the renal artery.

Extracellular accumulations
These are of little significance in chemically induced pathology, but assume some importance in the pathology of ageing animals. The major accumulations include hyaline degeneration, fibrinoid degeneration, amyloid degeneration and mucoid degeneration.

Hyaline degeneration does not denote any specific extracellular substance. It is merely a descriptive term meaning a glassy refractile appearance at autopsy.

Histologically the matrix in which the cells are embedded appears homogeneously eosinophilic, usually due to accumulation of some form of protein. Fibrinoid degeneration refers to the accumulation of proteins in the wall of blood vessels. This stains brightly eosinophilic and is composed largely of fibrin together with other serum proteins such as immunoglobulins. Extracellular deposition of serum proteins is also the basis of amyloid degeneration. In contrast to fibrinoid it is a pale eosinophilic substance and deposited around vessels and basement membranes rather than in the wall. Macroscopically, affected organs may be enlarged, and in severe cases the amyloid may be seen as greyish waxy deposits. Mucoid degeneration is most commonly seen in tumours. These may be epithelial tumours which secrete mucin or connective tissue tumours secreting mucopolysaccharides between the fibres. In these connective tissue tumours the term 'myxomatous' is often used to describe their gelatinous appearance.

Proliferation

In contrast to reduced growth, cytoplasmic accumulations or death, a cell may respond to chemical stress by increased growth at any structural level from the molecular to the cellular. Proliferations include a diverse range of responses from adaptive homeostasis to the irreversible proliferation of whole cell populations known as cancer. The two main descriptive terms for proliferations are hypertrophy and hyperplasia. Hypertrophy is an increase in size, hyperplasia an increase in numbers. There is considerable overlap in the use of these terms depending on the method used to examine the cells. For example, hyperplasia of subcellular organelles easily visible by electron microscopy may only be discernible by light microscopy as a general increase in cell size, namely, hypertrophy. Similarly, hyperplasia of whole cells through cell division may appear at necropsy as an enlarged or hypertrophied organ. This section will concentrate mainly on proliferation of organelles and of whole cells. The latter may be non-neoplastic or neoplastic.

Organelle proliferation

Many cell functions are dependent on the activity of specific organelles in the cell. Any demand on the cell to increase its functional activity may require proliferation of one or more organelles to satisfy the demand. Thus, organelle proliferation is often an adaptive homeostatic response rather than a true pathological change. However, if demand is excessive or prolonged, adaptation may fail and the cell is damaged. In principle almost any organelle could proliferate, but in practice chemically-induced SER, peroxisomal, mitochondrial and chromosome proliferations (polyploidy) are the ones most frequently detected (Figure 2.11). They usually result in cell enlargement, namely hypertrophy.

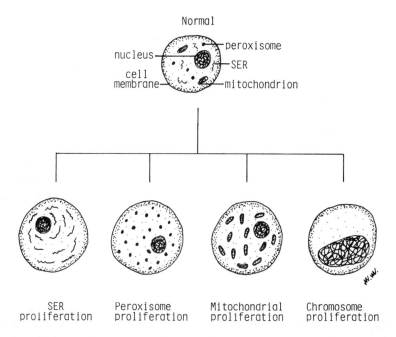

Figure 2.11. Examples of organelle proliferation in liver.

Smooth endoplasmic reticulum

SER (microsomal) proliferation is a common response to chemicals reaching the liver which is the major site of biotransformation of xenobiotics. Many of the biotransforming enzymes, such as the mono-oxygenase cytochrome P450, are associated with SER. Several chemicals have a non-polar region in the molecule which permits lipid solubility at physiological pH. Elimination of such molecules is more efficient if they are converted to more polar and more water-soluble substances by the xenobiotic metabolising enzymes. Continued exposure to xenobiotics may induce enzyme synthesis and proliferation of SER supporting the enzymes. This proliferation is most obvious ultrastructurally as an accumulation of smooth membranous profiles in the hepatocyte cytoplasm. This may not be detectable histologically, but in well-developed cases the cells are enlarged and the cytoplasm assumes a very fine pale vesicular or granular eosinophilic appearance.

Peroxisomes

Peroxisomes (microbodies) are a group of intracytoplasmic particles limited by a single membrane. They contain several enzyme systems associated, for example, with disposal of hydrogen peroxide and with the beta-oxidation of long-chain monounsaturated fatty acids. Chemically induced proliferation of peroxisomes is not common, but dramatic responses can occur in rodent liver cells following the administration of certain types of hypolipidaemics and plasticisers. These peroxisomes are too small to be seen by light microscopy, but the cytoplasm assumes a bright eosinophilia when there are large numbers in the cell.

Mitochondria

These are the key sites of the enzymes of the respiratory chain. A marked increase in mitochondria is not a common response to chemicals, but increases are sometimes seen. Marked increases give the cell a bright eosinophilic granularity. These mitochondria-rich cells are sometimes known as oncocytes. Oncocytes have been induced experimentally in the rat liver with antihistaminic methapyrilene, and in the collecting tubules of the rat kidney by the bipyridylium herbicide morfamquat. Other chemicals such as cuprizone cause enlargement of the mitochondria to produce megamitochondria.

DNA

Proliferation of chromosomal DNA may occur in the absence of cell division to produce a state known as polyploidy. Most normal mammalian cells contain a single set of chromosomes from each parent and are characteristically diploid (2n). Some tissues such as urinary bladder and liver contain cells with multiple chromosome complements such as 4n, 8n or 16n. This physiological polyploidy is quite normal. The chromosomes may be contained in a single nucleus, within multiple nuclei or by a combination of both possibilities. For example, binucleate cells may represent 30 % of hepatocytes in adult rodent liver, and individual nuclei with octaploid (8n) chromosomal content are by no means uncommon.

The degree of ploidy in a tissue may be increased by stimulating the division of physiologically polyploid cells or by an antimitotic effect inhibiting the cleavage of DNA synthesising cells. Liver necrosis, for example, will result in DNA synthesis in surviving hepatocytes some of which inevitably will be binucleate (2n + 2n). The end result of DNA replication of binucleate cells is a higher ploidy state such as two quadraploid (4n) daughter cells or a binucleate cell with quadraploid nuclei. Chronic liver damage with ongoing repair processes can thus lead to an insidious increase in cell ploidy recognised as an increase in cell and nuclear size. Other toxicants such as pyrrolizidine alkaloids interfere with mitosis and cell division. The hepatocytes may reduplicate their DNA in response to injury, but subsequently they are unable to divide. Eventually nuclei and cells become very large indeed and such cells have been called megalocytes.

Non-neoplastic proliferation (Figure 2.12)

Controlled, non-neoplastic cell proliferations include regeneration, hyperplasia, metaplasia and dysplasia. These may exist in pure form or overlap to varying degrees depending on the nature and extent of the inciting stimulus. Regeneration is the mechanism by which lethally injured cells are replaced and is considered in more detail in the section on inflammation and repair.

Hyperplasia

This generally refers to an absolute increase in the number of cells in a tissue or organ. It is conventionally divided into physiological and pathological categories. The proliferative response in the liver sometimes associated with chemicals causing SER proliferation is generally considered to be an adaptive or physiological hyperplasia. Hyperplasia of various uterine cells during the normal cycle is an example of a physiological hyperplasia that is commonly seen in endocrine-related tissue. Physiological hyperplasias are usually diffuse effects throughout the affected tissue or organ.

Pathological hyperplasias may affect tissues diffusely or in an irregular manner. Diffuse hyperplastic responses may be seen in epithelial cells subject to persistent low grade chronic irritation or to endocrine imbalance. In chronically irritated skin or bladder, the rate of epithelial cell proliferation increases to replace lost or damaged cells and if injury persists, the proliferation persists and the epithelium ultimately becomes thickened. In the skin, this thickening would be diagnosed as acanthosis, and in the bladder as urothelial hyperplasia. Pathological hyperplasias due to endocrine imbalance are common in ageing animals. For example, chronic endocrine imbalance due to pituitary or ovarian dysfunction is a frequent cause of endometrial hyperplasia in the uterus. Chemicals may also produce chronic endocrine imbalance, diffuse thyroid hyperplasia produced by goitrogens being a classic example.

The more problematical hyperplasias for the toxicological pathologist are those in which cell structure, growth, and organisation are not uniform. These range from proliferation of small groups of cells in otherwise normal organs (focal hyperplasia) to irregular nodular growths arising in a diffusely hyperplastic organ (diffuse nodular hyperplasia). Other variants include atypical hyperplasia, papillomatous hyperplasia and adenomatous hyperplasia, all of which indicate cells proliferating in a seemingly abnormal pattern. Since abnormal growth patterns are a feature of neoplasms the problem for the pathologist is to distinguish between non-neoplastic and neoplastic proliferations. This is one of the most difficult areas of decision making in pathology, even for the most experienced people, and accounts for the much-quoted expression, 'one man's hyperplasia is another man's neoplasia'. Because neoplasms sometimes arise in these areas of disorderly hyperplasia, such proliferations are often referred to as preneoplastic lesions.

Metaplasia

Metaplasia is a proliferation in which one type of differentiated cell is substituted for another type of differentiated cell. The change is commonly seen in lining epithelia, particularly in the respiratory and reproductive tract, but also occurs in connective tissue. In epithelia, it is usually associated with chronic irritation or endocrine imbalance and often takes the form of substitution of a columnar mucus-secreting surface by a stratified squamous epithelial surface. There is frequently an associated hyperplasia. Teleologically, metaplasia can usually be considered an adaptive response of an epithelium to an adverse environment and most often it is an orderly process resulting in a typical normal-appearing squamous epithelium. Sometimes, if there is persistent chronic injury, metaplastic change may become disorderly with variations in cell size, orientation and staining properties. This is termed atypical squamous metaplasia. In the bronchial epithelium of cigarette smokers it is a frequent precursor of bronchial neoplasms. Thus, the significance of metaplasia can range from a simple adaptive response to a preneoplastic change and the pathologist is faced with the same diagnostic problems as with the interpretation of hyperplasia.

Dysplasia

This is the most disorderly of the non-neoplastic proliferations. It often accompanies hyperplasia and metaplasia and consists of increased mitotic activity producing excess cells of various shapes, sizes and degrees of differentiation arranged in a disorderly architectural pattern. Nuclear abnormalities such as variable degrees of ploidy and abnormal mitotic figures are prominent features. Like the other forms of non-neoplastic proliferations it is commonly associated with chronic irritation or endocrine imbalance. Dysplasia is a reversible proliferation, but in the more extreme cases the cellular abnormalities approach those seen in neoplastic growths.

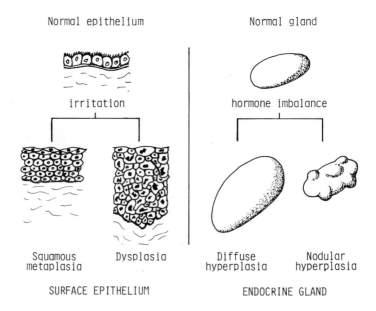

Figure 2.12. Examples of non-neoplastic cell proliferations.

Neoplastic proliferation

Cell proliferations that show partial or complete loss of responsiveness to normal growth controls are termed neoplasms. The mechanisms by which chemicals may lead to uncontrolled cell proliferation are outside the scope of this book, but they essentially fall into the same two mechanistic categories as other forms of toxicity. For example, chemicals may act intracellularly, particularly on DNA (genotoxic carcinogens), or may modify dietary, hormonal or other regulatory factors in the extracellular environment (non-genotoxic carcinogens). Attention is focused on the principles of morphological classification of neoplasms. The essential component of the definition of neoplasia is lack of responsiveness to growth control or 'autonomy'. It is this autonomy that distinguishes neoplasia from reversible processes such as hyperplasia and metaplasia. Unfortunately, autonomy is often difficult to prove and has to be assumed on the basis of other more easily identifiable characteristics. These characteristics include evidence of structural, biochemical and behavioural atypia amongst the proliferating cells. Some of these are listed in Table 2.1.

Table 2.1. Some features of autonomous proliferations.

Structural atypia	Biochemical atypia	Behavioural atypia
Pleomorphism	Abnormal secretion	Increased mitosis
Cytomegaly	Abnormal enzymes	Loss of cell contact
Basophilia	Abnormal antigens	Compressing adjacent tissue
Disorganisation	Abnormal storage	Invasion

Benign and malignant classification

Autonomous proliferations are classified into two important categories — benign and malignant. This classification is based primarily on whether cell proliferation remains localised to the site of origin or whether it is likely to spread (metastasise) to other sites. The propensity to remain localised or to spread elsewhere is often correlated with certain morphological characteristics. These characteristics are the cornerstones of the pathologist's diagnosis. At necropsy, benign neoplasms are well circumscribed, often encapsulated, growths that compress the surrounding tissue. Malignant tumours are irregular, ill-defined, non-encapsulated growths which invade and destroy the surrounding normal tissue and ultimately produce metastatic growths in other sites (Figure 2.13).

Histological criteria for distinguishing benign and malignant neoplasms are based mainly on cell structure, organisation and mitotic activity. The cells of benign neoplasms resemble their cells of origin, show a remarkable uniformity in cell size, shape and nuclear configuration, and are organised into structures which mimic that of their parent organ. They have relatively infrequent mitotic

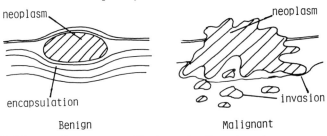

Figure 2.13. Macroscopic appearance of benign and malignant neoplasms.

figures which is consistent with the slow rate of growth of these neoplasms. The boundary between the neoplastic and normal cells is well demarcated and may take the form of a fibrous capsule. At the other extreme, highly malignant cells bear little resemblance to their cell of origin (anaplasia), vary widely in size, shape and nuclear configuration (pleomorphism) and are disorganised. Mitotic figures are frequent and sometimes abnormal. Although the great majority of neoplasms can be classified as benign or malignant using these criteria, it should be stressed that some neoplasms fall into an intermediate grey area and cannot be classified with certainty. This uncertainty and that involved in distinguishing hyperplasia from neoplasia is a significant problem in toxicological pathology, particularly in long-term bioassays in rodents where precise classifications may be required for statistical analyses of data.

Histogenetic classification

The second categorisation in the diagnosis of neoplasms is the cell and tissue of origin of the proliferation. At a very basic level, neoplasms may arise from epithelial tissues and mesenchymal tissues. Benign tumours in both epithelial and mesenchymal tissues are generally designated by the suffix -oma. Malignant tumours are designated -carcinoma when they arise in epithelial tissues and -sarcoma if they have a mesenchymal origin. In addition, a prefix or a preceding word is often used to specify the precise origin and structure of the neoplasm. The following are a few examples of histogenetic classification.

Benign epithelial neoplasms are essentially of two types, papillomas and adenomas (Figure 2.14). Papillomas arise from surface epithelium such as the epidermis. As the epithelium proliferates it is thrown into finger-like projections supported by blood vessels and connective tissue. Adenomas are proliferations of glandular epithelium and of epithelium forming solid organs such as the liver. Additional qualifying terms are often used to describe certain architectural features of the neoplasm or to specify the cell or origin or nature of the epithelium. For example, an adenoma may contain large cystic structures and the term cystadenoma could be used to indicate this feature. Similarly, a papilloma arising in the skin may be described as squamous to indicate the type of epithelium affected, and adenomas in the thyroid are qualified as follicular cell or C-cell to specify the cell of origin.

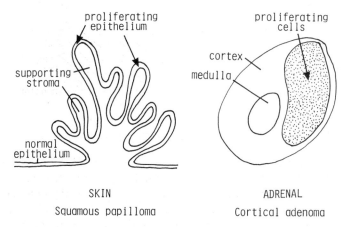

Figure 2.14. Examples of benign epithelial neoplasms.

Carcinomas are malignant epithelial neoplasms. This diagnosis is often qualified to indicate other features of the tumour such as cell type or organisation. Squamous carcinoma and adenocarcinoma are two of the most frequently used diagnoses. If the cells are so rapidly dividing that they do not differentiate into cells of recognisable origin they are termed anaplastic carcinomas.

The nomenclature for benign mesenchymal tumours is generally straight-forward. The suffix -oma is combined with a prefix designating the cell or tissue of origin. For example benign tumours of bone, fat and fibrous tissues are osteoma, lipoma and fibroma respectively. Their malignant counterparts are designated by the suffix -sarcoma — namely, osteosarcoma, liposarcoma and fibrosarcoma. Unfortunately, there are exceptions to the rules and some '-omas' such as melanoma and mesothelioma in man are malignant proliferations.

The nomenclature also has to cover situations in which two or more cell types appear to be proliferating. This is often encountered in the mammary gland. In the rat, both fibrous tissue and glandular epithelial components frequently show marked proliferation and the neoplasm is diagnosed as a fibroadenoma. More bizarre combinations such as bone, cartilage, fibrous and glandular tissue occur in mammary tumours of the bitch and these are simply termed mixed mammary tumours or complex adenoma.

Other classifications

In addition to the classifications discussed above, pathologists frequently use further qualifying or quantifying terms to classify neoplasms in more detail. Neoplastic proliferation is a long-term process in which a cell or group of cells gradually develops from a microscopic entity to a grossly visible mass. The most important classifying terms are those that state the level of development of the neoplasm. The main terminologies are staging and grading. Staging is a clinical assessment by a physician or surgeon of the degree of spread of malignant disease.

It is based on the size of the primary lesion, its extent of spread to regional lymph nodes and the presence or absence of metastases. It usually comprises a 3–5 point scale in which stage 1 refers to a small local growth and the higher stages indicate progressively disseminated widespread disease.

Grading is the method used by pathologists to classify the stage of development or degree of malignancy of a neoplasm. There are various ways of grading, but they usually include an assessment of the cytology of the individual cells, the size of the growth, or a combination of both parameters. For example, Broder's grading of squamous cell carcinoma in man ranges from well differentiated slowly dividing tumour cells to poorly differentiated tumour cells with frequent mitoses. Grading is also an important consideration in toxicological pathology. For example, tumours may be graded on the basis of size from microscopic to macroscopic growths, or on the basis of their extension beyond local anatomical boundaries such as a muscle layer. A form of grading important in some forms of statistical analysis (Chapter 5) is grading tumours as incidental or fatal. Incidental tumours are those found in animals dying from other causes and fatal tumours are ones leading to illness or death of the animal.

Finally, the classification of neoplasia has to take into account that carcinogenesis is a multistage process and the morphological expression of the process is also multistage. The administration of carcinogenic chemicals leads to a spectrum of proliferations, and the nature of the spectrum varies according to the rate and extent of exposure. For example, the sequential analysis of liver after different periods of carcinogen administration often reveals microscopic proliferations of altered liver cells in the first few weeks followed by larger nodular growths and eventually by atypical growths that are unequivocally cancer. The various stages in this process of neoplastic transformation in the liver are classified as foci, areas, nodules and carcinoma, but the point in the spectrum at which autonomous growth begins cannot be determined. If treatment is withdrawn during the first few weeks, many of the foci and nodules will regress, but a minority of seemingly identical proliferations may progress as autonomous growths. Currently, there are no consistent morphological markers to identify cells in the early stages of autonomous growth. This returns us to the problem of differentiating hyperplasia from neoplasia which pervades the classification of proliferations in toxicological pathology.

Inflammation and repair

Degeneration and proliferation are the main cellular responses to injury, but these are frequently accompanied by an extracellular response to contain or remove the injurious agent and repair the damaged tissue. These extracellular processes which follow cell and tissue injury are termed inflammation and repair. Inflammation is a dynamic process, the extent and nature of which varies according to the nature, extent and duration of injury. It includes vascular, neurological, humoral and cellular responses at the site of injury. It is conventionally divided into acute and chronic inflammation. Repair is also a dynamic process and consists of two main elements, regeneration and fibrosis. Inflammation and repair frequently occur together and in some conditions, such as persistent injury, acute and chronic inflammation, regeneration and fibrosis may occur simultaneously. For convenience, each element will be described separately.

Acute inflammation

This is the immediate and early response to an injurious agent and affects the vascular and connective tissues adjacent to the injured cells. There are three major components in the process of acute inflammation: increased blood flow (vasodilation), increased vascular permeability (exudation) and egress of white blood cells into the injured tissue (emigration). These three components are coordinated and interrelated by numerous chemical mediators produced or released at the site of injury. Mediators include histamine, bradykinin, complement and many other pharmacologically active substances. The emphasis in this section is on the morphological aspects of the inflammatory process visible to the pathologist (Figure 2.15) rather than on the pharmacological and biochemical events.

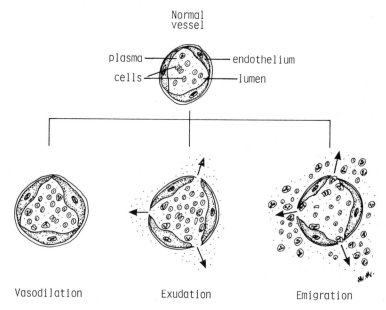

Figure 2.15. Major components of acute inflammation.

Vasodilation

Vaso dilation occurs directly after injury. The microvasculature at the site of injury becomes dilated and filled with blood (hyperaemia). Blood flow through the dilated microvasculature is initially rapid, but soon slows because a concomitant increase in vascular permeability and loss of plasma water raises the viscosity of the blood. In the slowly moving blood the pattern of flow changes. Red cells tend to clump in the centre of the vessel lumen and leucocytes assume a more peripheral position near the vessel wall. This margination of leucocytes is an important initial step in the emigration process. If flow becomes very slow, the blood may clot and form a thrombus.

Exudation

This is the increased passage of fluid and solutes, notably proteins, through the vessel wall. The mechanisms leading to increased vascular permeability are complex and incompletely understood. They include endothelial cell contraction or damage, the effects of mediators, local haemodynamic forces and the osmotic effects of proteins escaping into interstitial tissue. The leak of proteins is roughly in proportion to their molecular size. Albumin is in the greatest amount, but if vascular permeability is extensive, large amounts fibrinogen may leak out. Exudation is an important local defence mechanism. The increase in interstitial fluid dilutes toxins, and proteins such as globulins are effective in neutralising agents like bacteria. This increased fluid is sometimes called inflammatory oedema or simply oedema.

Emigration

Emigration of white blood cells, principally neutrophils and monocytes is also an important defence mechanism. These are phagocytic cells which engulf and digest foreign particulate matter such as bacteria and the debris of dead cells. The emigration of leucocytes is an active process which occurs in two stages. The cells stick to the endothelial surface (pavementing) and then actively migrate through the gaps between the endothelial cells and into the tissue spaces. The mechanism by which leucocytes stick to the endothelial cells is unknown. Emigration is an active amoeboid process and once outside the vessel, neutrophils can move as fast as 20 μm per minute. Monocytes, which differentiate into macrophages, move more slowly. Movement of leucocytes in tissue spaces is polarised in the general direction of the site of injury. This process, known as chemotaxis, is mediated by various chemical attractants such as components of the complement, kinin and clotting systems. Because neutrophils are in greater number in the circulating blood and because they move faster than macrophages, the first phase of cellular infiltration into damaged tissue is dominated by neutrophils. With the passage of time, macrophage numbers increase and after 2 or 3 days macrophages outnumber neutrophils in most inflammations. In addition to leucocyte emigration, red cells may burst through the vessel wall behind an exiting white cell. This is a passive movement in contrast to energy-dependent white cell emigration and is termed diapedesis ('to walk between').

Variants

Whilst the major components of acute inflammation are present in all damaged tissue, the proportions vary according to the nature, duration and extent of injury and to the nature of the injured tissue itself. Qualifying terms may be used to specify the dominant features of the inflammation (Figure 2.16). For example, serous exudate refers to the fluid-filled blister after burns. Fibrinous exudate occurs in the peritoneal cavity of rats given ulcerogenic non-steroidal anti-inflammatories, and haemorrhagic inflammation is a common local perivascular reaction to irritants injected intravenously. Excess mucous secretion in an inflamed epithelium, such as the nose in common colds, is termed catarrhal inflammation.

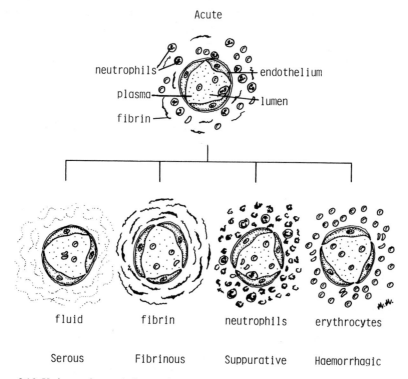

Figure 2.16. Variants of acute inflammation.

Sequelae (Figure 2.17)

Acute inflammation is the first step in a dynamic response to injury. The sequelae depend on the nature and extent of injury. Resolution means the complete restoration of normal conditions after the cause of the acute inflammation is removed. This occurs when there is minimal cell death and tissue damage, rapid elimination of the causal agent, and local conditions favouring the removal of fluid and debris by lymphatics and by phagocytosis.

Organisation is the deposition of fibrous tissue in inflamed areas. It occurs when there is excessive exudate or necrosis and when local conditions are unfavourable for the removal of exudate and debris. It is common after fibrinous inflammation. Fibrin deposits in some sites, such as on the pleura of inflamed lungs, are not easily removed. Capillaries grow into the fibrin strands and the fibrin is gradually replaced by collagen produced by the fibroblasts which accompany the ingrowing capillaries. This fibrous tissue may eventually join two adjacent surfaces to form an adhesion. Deposition of fibrous tissue to fill the gap left by dead tissue is also part of the repair process.

An abscess is one sequel to suppurative inflammation. Suppurative inflammation is characterised by tissue damage and an intense prolonged neutrophil emigration. It is seen, for example, in skin injected with irritant chemicals such as turpentine. The neutrophils die and liquefy and together with the liquefied dead tissue form a purulent exudate (pus). The pus is walled-off from the surrounding tissue by fibrous tissue to form an abscess, which may subsequently burst and heal. Finally, the causal agent may persist and with it the inflammatory process, but in an altered form. The continuing process is known as chronic inflammation.

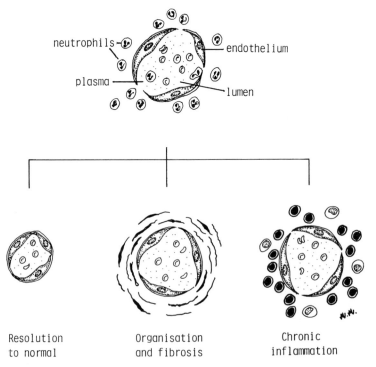

Figure 2.17. Sequelae to acute inflammation.

Chronic inflammation

This may be a sequel to acute inflammation if the causal agent persists or is repeatedly applied. Chronic inflammation may also occur as a primary process if the injurious agent is of low toxicity. For example, continued inhalation of silica may initiate a chronic inflammatory reaction in the lung, termed silicosis, without any initial acute response. In contrast to the neutrophil-rich exudate of acute inflammation, chronic inflammation is characterised by the accumulation or proliferation of mononuclear leucocytes, vascular endothelium and fibroblasts (Figure 2.18).

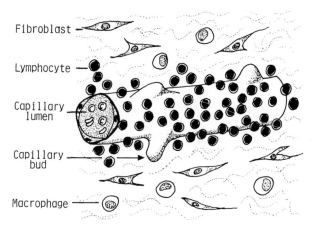

Figure 2.18. Major components of chronic inflammation.

The two main mononuclear leucocytes are macrophages (histiocytes) and lymphoid cells such as lymphocytes and plasma cells. Macrophages are the major phagocytic cells of chronic inflammatory reactions. They are derived from blood monocytes and also proliferate locally. Macrophages move more slowly than neutrophils, but they can survive for long periods in contrast to the short-lived neutrophils. They digest cell debris and other particulate material such as bacteria. In response to certain injurious agents, notably those that are difficult to digest because of their size or composition, macrophages may enlarge to form pale epithelial-like cells (epithelioid cells) or may fuse to form large cells with multiple nuclei known as giant cells. Lymphoid cells are also common in most forms of chronic inflammation. These reflect the body's immune response to foreign antigens or to endogenous molecules altered as a result of cell injury. Proliferation of capillaries and fibroblasts is an attempt to wall off the damage or to repair the damaged area. Tissue rich in fibroblasts and capillaries is termed granulation tissue.

Variants

There is considerable variation in the proportions of these major components

Principles of Toxicological Pathology

depending on the nature, intensity and persistence of the causal agent (Figure 2.19). Chronic inflammation is frequently sub-classified accordingly. Chronic lymphocytic inflammation is usually associated with persistent antigenic stimulation as in autoimmune diseases. Persistence of an indigestible agent such as Mycobacteria species or injected oily substances may produce a chronic histiocytic reaction. These histiocyte-rich responses are often referred to as granulomas or granulomatous inflammation. Fibroblastic and vascular proliferation often dominate the chronic reaction to persistent irritation or trauma.

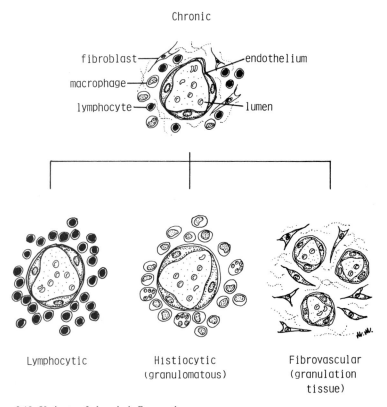

Figure 2.19. Variants of chronic inflammation.

Repair by regeneration

Regeneration is one of the two basic ways in which dead cells are replaced by viable cells. The other is by fibrosis. In regeneration, the replacement cells are of the same type as those that were damaged. For example, dead liver cells may be replaced by proliferation of adjacent healthy liver cells. In the early phases of regeneration the proliferating cells are undifferentiated and appear basophilic. In some tissues such as the kidney, these basophilic cells are often in striking contrast to the normally eosinophilic epithelial cells. Eventually, the cells differentiate to the normal functional state. The degree of regeneration depends on the nature and persistence of the injury. If injury persists, proliferation persists to balance continuing cell loss. Ultimately this results in an increased number of cells in the injured organ. This is a form of hyperplasia.

The capacity to regenerate is related to the amount of proliferation and replacement that normally takes place in the organ. Some cells, such as those lining the intestinal tract, proliferate throughout life and their regenerative capacity is enormous. Other tissues are composed of stable cells which do not actively replicate under normal circumstances, but which retain the latent capacity to proliferate in response to damage. For example, mitotic figures are rare in adult liver, but cells will proliferate rapidly if part of the liver is removed or damaged. Finally, some tissues contain permanent cells which are unable to multiply. Cells such as neurons and heart muscle cannot regenerate and damage has to be repaired by other means. This is repair by fibrosis.

The perfection of parenchymal repair depends not only on the ability of cells to regenerate, but on the integrity of the tissue supporting the cells. A toxin such as mercuric chloride may destroy renal tubular cells without damaging the tubular basement membrane or underlying stroma. Regeneration from surviving tubular cells may completely restore normal structure and function. Regeneration on a damaged stroma may result in an imperfect structure. If all tubular epithelial cells are destroyed, regeneration is impossible and the area is repaired by fibrosis (Figure 2.20).

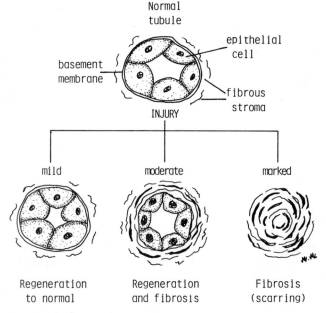

Figure 2.20. Repair of renal tubular injury.

Repair by fibrosis

Fibrosis has been mentioned several times and emphasises the overlap and integration of many of the processes of inflammation and repair. With the exception of minor damage restricted to epithelial surfaces, most tissue injuries include the underlying supporting connective tissue stroma. When injury is slight, the connective-tissue elements may also undergo healing by regeneration. When the damage is more severe, and particularly when the specialised epithelial or parenchymal cells fail to regenerate adequately, the gap is filled by the formation of a new connective tissue (granulation tissue). In the early stages of connective-tissue repair new capillary-size blood vessels and plump active fibroblasts derived from the adjacent healthy connective tissue proliferate and actively grow into the gap. The initial granulation tissue is highly vascular and cellular, but as the fibroblasts secrete more and more collagen precursors the subsequent collagen formation dominates the area. The fibroblasts eventually become inactive and revert to fibrocytes and as the collagen matures the area contracts to form a scar. Scarring is an inevitable consequence of all repair except for the ideal situation in which a simple parenchymal injury permits perfect regeneration and reconstitution of the original architecture.

Summary

The response of cells and tissues to injury is limited. Intracellular or extracellular injury results in either degeneration or proliferation in the affected cells and is frequently accompanied by the processes of inflammation and repair. These are all dynamic processes and can occur in a variety of combinations depending on the nature of the chemical, its potency and the duration of exposure. Commonly encountered responses related to the two important characteristics, potency and duration, are illustrated in Figure 2.21. In the following chapter this basic theme is applied to some of the more commonly encountered examples of target organ pathology. However, before doing this, it is important to look at the way the language of pathology is constructed around this theme and at some of the important qualifying terminology that is used to put the theme into context in toxicology.

The language of pathology

The vocabulary and construction of the language of pathology often forms a barrier to communication. They may sometimes cause serious problems in the dialogue between pathologists and toxicologists or other interested parties such as regulatory and consumer bodies. A brief account of the construction of the language should help the reader to understand some of the descriptive pathology in Chapters 3 and 4. Unfortunately, the vocabulary has to be learned in the same way as in any other language, by experience and by reference to dictionaries.

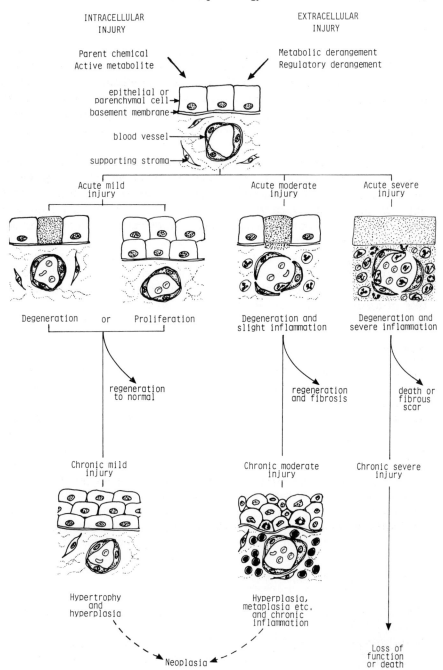

Figure 2.21. Common mechanisms and responses to injury.

Much of the language is built around the principle of cause and effect and is based on the mechanisms and responses to injury described earlier in this chapter. The aim is to convey concisely the observations that the pathologist has made. Since most of the observations are of abnormal responses in tissues and cells most of the vocabulary is designed to describe effects rather than causal mechanisms. There are two major components in any description of effects: the location of the effect and its nature. These two major components may be accompanied by a variety of qualifying words used to define the location and nature of the effect more precisely.

The two main components, location and effect, may be presented either as separate words or be combined into a single word in which the prefix designates the location and the suffix the type of process. The location, for example an organ or tissue, may be designated by its 'common' name when used as a noun or by a latin derivation when used in the adjectival or prefix form. Thus, a degeneration such as cell death in the liver may be termed either liver necrosis or hepatic necrosis, and inflammation (suffix -itis) of the liver may be termed in the combined form as the single word hepatitis. The student unfortunately has little choice but to try to become familiar with the more common terms and combining forms that are used in pathology. Many of these have already been used in this chapter but a few more examples of component forms are presented in Table 2.2.

Table 2.2.   Examples of combining forms used in diagnoses.

Organ	Prefix	Process	Suffix
Liver	Hepat-	Degeneration	-osis/-opathy
Kidney	Nephr-	Inflammation	-itis
Joint	Arthr-	Proliferation	-plasia/-oma

Qualifying terms are often used to specify the location or to define the nature of the process more precisely. Thus, inflammation in the kidney may be diagnosed as nephritis, or more precisely as tubular nephritis if the inflammatory process is located in the tubules rather than in the glomeruli. Similarly, inflammation is a dynamic process with many phases and the phase may be specified by use of such terms as acute and chronic. Acute tubular nephritis is thus a more precise diagnosis than just nephritis.

It is very important in toxicological pathology to qualify the diagnosis in a way that indicates the effect of the pathological process on the normal structure and functioning of the organ. Not only do we need to know the type of pathological process that is present and its location, but we need to know whether it is of minor or major significance to the function of that organ. Two main groups of qualifiers are used to convey this significance. They are known as distribution terms and severity (or grade) terms. The main terms are listed in Table 2.3. Distribution terms are used to define the way the effect is spread across the organ or tissue.

Table 2.3. Common qualifying terms used to assess the effect of the pathological process on organ function.

Distribution	Severity
Unilateral	Minimal
Bilateral	Slight
Focal	Moderate
Multifocal	Marked
Diffuse	Severe

This ranges from a single small locus (focal) to involvement of the entire organ (diffuse). Involvement of paired organs such as the kidney may be specified as unilateral or bilateral depending on whether one or both organs are involved. The severity terms are self-explanatory and range from minor to major degrees of effect.

An acute tubular nephritis may thus be considered of minor significance if qualified as focal and slight and of major significance if described as diffuse and severe. This 'biological significance' or 'biological valency' assigned to the pathological process may be of considerable importance in data interpretation. For example, designation of tumours as lethal or incidental is required for certain statistical analyses of tumour data.

Another important point related to diagnoses and data interpretation is the relative factual value of any diagnosis. A gastric ulcer has well-defined diagnostic criteria and can be reasonably considered to be a factual diagnosis by a competent pathologist. However, in some areas of pathology, the criteria for arriving at a particular diagnosis are less well defined and the diagnosis may be little more than an opinion that the process observed lies in a particular spectrum or range. 'One man's hyperplasia is another man's neoplasia' has already been mentioned. It is this point that is particularly difficult to portray to non-pathologists, and it is also a point that is sometimes forgotten by pathologists themselves.

Finally, a pathologist may include a statement about the cause (aetiology) of the effect he observes. For example, an inflammation in the lung may be diagnosed as pneumonia, but if viral inclusions can be identified in the tissue the diagnosis would be extended to viral pneumonia to incorporate a statement about the cause of the process. Similarly, a nematode worm migrating through tissue may incite a granulomatous inflammation. If the worm is still visible histologically, the term parasitic or verminous granuloma will be a more informative diagnosis than just granuloma. Unfortunately, chemicals, other than those in particulate or fibrous forms, are not visible by conventional pathological techniques and a pathologist is restricted to the diagnosis of effects. Statements or inferences about the cause are derived by judgements using other means such as statistical analysis (Chapter 5) or the biological consistency of the observed response with hypotheses of possible intracellular or extracellular mechanisms of chemical injury.

Bibliography

General toxicology and mechanisms of injury

Albert, A. (1979) *Selective Toxicity.* (London: Chapman and Hall)

Aldridge, W. N. (1981) Mechanisms of toxicity: New concepts are required in toxicology. *Trends Pharmacol. Sci.*, 2: 228

Ariens, E. J., Simonis, A. M. and Offermerer, J. (1976) *Introduction to General Toxicology,* (New York: Academic Press)

Arnott, M. S., Vaneys, J. and Wang, Y. M. (1982) *Molecular Interrelations of Nutrition and Cancer.* (New York: Raven Press)

Bhatnagar, R. S. (ed.) (1980) *Molecular Basis of Environmental Toxicity.* (Ann Arbor: Ann Arbor Science Publications)

Boyd, M. R. (1980) Biochemical mechanisms in chemical induced lung injury: roles of metabolic activation. *CRC Crit. Rev. Toxicol.*, 7: 103.

Bridges, J. W., Benford, D. J. and Hubbard, S. A. (1983) Mechanisms of toxic injury. In *Celluar Systems for Toxicity Testing*, edited by G. M. Williams, V. C. Dunkel and V. A. Ray (New York: New York Academy of Sciences)

Bus, J. S. and Gibson, J. E. (1979) Lipid peroxidation and its role in toxicology. In *Reviews in Biochemical Toxicology*, Vol. 1, edited by E. Hodgson, J. R. Bend and R. M. Philpot (New York: Elsevier-North Holland)

Bus, J. S. and Gibson, J.E. (1982–83) Mechanisms of superoxide radical-mediated toxicity. *J. Toxicol. Clin. Toxicol.*, 19: 689.

Carroll, K. K. (1980) Lipids and carcinogenesis. *J. Environ. Pathol. Toxicol.*, 3: 253.

Chambers, P. L. and Gunsel, P. (eds.) (1979) Mechanisms of toxic action on some target organs. *Archs. Toxicol.*, Suppl. 2.

Cowley, R. A. and Trump, B. F. *Pathophysiology of Shock, Anoxia, and Ischemia.* (Baltimore: Williams & Wilkins)

Doull, J., Klaassen, C. D. and Amdur, M. O. (eds.) (1980) *Casarett and Doull's Toxicology, The Basic Science of Poisons.* (New York: Macmillan)

Eichler, O. (ed.) (1976) *Experimental Production of Disease.* (Berlin: Springer-Verlag)

Ferguson, G. G. (1984) *Pathophysiology: Mechanisms and Expressions.* (London: W. B. Saunders)

Fortmeyer, H. P. (1982) The influence of exogenous factors such as maintenance and nutrition on the course and results of animal experiments. In *Animals in Toxicological Research*, edited by I. Bartosek, A. Guaitani and E. Pacei (New York: Raven Press)

Gibson, G. G., Hubbard, R. and Parke, D. V. (1983) *Immunotoxicology.* (London: Academic Press)

Gillette, J. R. and Pohl, L. R. (1977) A prospective on covalent binding and toxicity. *J. Toxicol. Environ. Health*, 2: 849.

Gillette, J. R. (1980) An overview of the role of microsomal enzymes in the formation of toxic metabolites. In *Microsomes, Drug Oxidations and Chemical Carcinogenesis*, (London: Academic Press)

Goldstein, A., Aronow, L. and Kalman, S. M. (1974) *Principles of Drug Action: The Basis of Pharmacology.* (New York: John Wiley)

Goldstein, D. B. (1984) The effects of drugs on membrane fluidity. *Ann. Rev. Pharmacol. Toxicol.*, 24: 43.

Gorrod, J. W. (ed.) (1979) *Drug Toxicity.* (London: Taylor and Francis)

Gorrod, J. W. (1981) Covalent binding as an indicator of drug toxicity. In *Testing for Toxicity*, edited by J. W. Gorrod (London: Taylor and Francis)

Hayes A. W. (ed.) (1982) *Principles and Methods of Toxicology.* (New York: Raven Press)

Hodgson, E. and Guthrie, F. E. (eds.) (1980) *Introduction to Biochemical Toxicology.* (New York: Elsevier-North Holland)

General pathology49

General pathology

Hokama, Y. and Nakamura, R. M. (eds.) (1982) *Immunology and Immunopathology. Basic Concepts.* (Boston: Little, Brown)

Homburger, F., Hayes, J. A. and Pelikan, E. W. (eds.) (1983) *A Guide to General Toxicology.* (Basel: Karger)

Hook, J. B., McCormack, K. M. and Kluwe, W. M. (1979) Biochemical mechanisms of nephrotoxicity. In *Reviews in Biochemical Toxicology*, Vol. 1, edited by E. Hodgson, J. R. Bend and R. M. Philpot (New York: Elsevier-North Holland)

Jakoby, W. B., Bend, J. R. and Caldwell, J. (eds.) (1982) *Metabolic Basic of Detoxification: Metabolism of Functional Groups.* (New York: Academic Press)

Loomis, T. A. (1978) *Essentials of Toxicology.* (Philadelphia: Lea & Febiger)

Miller, M. J. (1983) *Pathophysiology: Principles of Disease.* (London: W. B. Saunders)

Mitchell, J. R., Hughes, H., Lauterburg, B. H. and Smith, C. V. (1982) Chemical nature of reactive intermediates as determinant of toxicologic responses. *Drug Metabol. Rev.*, 13: 539.

Mitchell, J. R. and Horning, M. J. (1984) *Drug Metabolism and Drug Toxicity.* (New York: Raven Press)

Oishi, S., Oishi, H. and Hiraga, K. (1979) The effect of food restriction for 4 weeks on common toxicity parameters in male rats. *Toxicol. Appl. Pharmacol.*, 47: 15.

Parke, D. V. (1968) *The Biochemistry of Foreign Compounds.* (Oxford: Pergamon)

Parke, D. V. (1982) Mechanisms of chemical toxicity — a unifying hypothesis. *Reg. Toxicol. Pharmacol.*, 2: 267.

Peters, R. A. (1963) *Biochemical Lesions and Lethal Synthesis.* (Oxford: Pergamon Press)

Roe, D. A. (ed.) (1983) *Diet, Nutrition and Cancer: From Basic Research to Policy Implications.* (New York: Liss)

Ross, M. H., Lustbader, E. D. and Bras, G. (1983). Bodyweight, dietary practices, and tumor susceptibility in the rat. *J. Nat. Cancer Inst.*, 71: 1041.

Sharma, R. P. and Street, J. C. (eds.) (1981) *Immunologic Considerations in Toxicology*, Vol. 1 and 2. (Boca Raton: CRC Press)

Slater, T. F. (ed.) (1978) *Biochemical Mechanisms of Liver Injury.* (London: Academic Press)

Smith, D. A. (ed.) (1977) Mechanisms of molecular and cellular toxicology. *J. Toxicol. Environ. Health*, 2: 1229.

Snyder, R., Parke, D. V., Kocsis, J., Jollow, D. J. and Gibson, C. G. (eds.) (1981) *Biological Reactive Intermediates 2: Chemical Mechanisms and Biological Effects.* (New York: Plenum Press)

Theofilopoulos, A. N. and Dixon, F. J. (1982) Autoimmune diseases: immunopathology and etiopathogenesis. *Am. J. Pathol.*, 108: 319.

Timbrell, J. A. (1982) *Principles of Biochemical Toxicology.* (London: Taylor and Francis)

Weck, A. L. D. and Bundgaard, H. (eds.) (1983) *Allergic Reactions to Drugs.* (Berlin: Springer-Verlag)

Yu, B. P., Masoro, E. J., Murata, I., Bertrand, H. A. and Lynd, F. T. (1982) Lifespan study of SPF Fischer-344 male rats fed ad-libitum or restricted diets — longevity, growth, lean body mass and disease. *J. Gerontol.*, 37: 130.

General pathology and responses to injury

Anderson, J. R. (ed.) (1980) *Muir's Textbook of Pathology.* (London: Arnold)

Bowen, I. D. and Lockshin, R. A. (1981) *Cell Death.* (London: Chapman and Hall)

Cohen, A. J. and Grasso, P. (1981) Review of hepatic response to hypolipidaemic drugs and assessment of its toxicological significance to man. *Fd. Cosmet. Toxicol.*, 19: 585.

Constantinides, P. (1984) *Ultrastructural Pathobiology.* (Amsterdam: Elsevier)

Farber, E. (1982) Sequential events in chemical carcinogenesis. In *Cancer, a Comprehensive Treatise. Vol. 1, Etiology: Chemical and Physical Carcinogenesis*, edited by F. F. Becker (New York: Plenum Press)

Foulds, L. (1969) *Neoplastic Development*, Vol. 1 (New York: Academic Press)

Gedigk, P. and Totovic, P. (1983) Lysosomes and lipopigments. In *Cellular Pathobiology of Human Disease*, edited by B. F. Trump, R.J. Jones and A. Laufer (New York: Gustav Fischer)

Govan, A. D. T. Macfarlane, P. S., and Callander, R. (1981) *Pathology Illustrated*. (Edinburgh: Churchill Livingstone)

Glynn, L. E. (ed.) (1981) *Tissue Repair and Regeneration*. (Amsterdam: Elsevier-North Holland)

Hartoft, W. S. (1972) Observation and interpretation of lipid pigments (lipofuscins) in the pathology of laboratory animals. *CRC Crit. Rev. Toxicol.*, 1: 379.

Kindl, H. and Lazarow, P. B. (eds.) (1982) *Peroxisomes and Glycoxysomes*. (New York: New York Academy of Science)

Kisilevsky, R. (1983) Amyloidosis: a familiar problem in the light of current pathogenetic developments. *Lab. Invest.*, 49: 381.

Majno, G., Lagattuta, M. and Thompson, T. (1960) Cellular death and necrosis; chemical, physical and morphological changes in rat liver. *Virchow. Arch. (Pathol. Anat.)*, 333: 421.

Mori, M. (1983) Ultrastructural changes of hepatocyte organelles induced by chemicals and their relation to fat accummulation in the liver. *Acta. Pathol. Jap.*, 33: 911.

Pitot, H. C. (1981). *Fundamentals of Oncology*. (New York: Marcel Dekker)

Reddy, J. K. and Lalwai, N. D. (1984) Carcinogenesis by hepatic peroxisome proliferators: evaluation of the risk of hypolipidermic drugs and industrial plasticizers to humans. *CRC Crit. Rev. Toxicol.*, 12: 1.

Reide, U. and Moore, G. W. (1983) Quantitative pathology by means of symbolic logic. *CRC Crit. Rev. Toxicol.*, 11: 279.

Ryan, G. B. and Majno, G. (1977) *Inflammation*. (Kalamazoo: Upjohn)

Spector, W. G. (1980) *An Introduction to General Pathology*. (Edinburgh: Churchill Livingstone)

Taussig, J. J. (1984) *Processes in Pathology and Microbiology*. (Oxford: Blackwell)

Trump, B. F., McDowell, E. M. and Arstila, A. U. (1980) Cellular reaction to injury. In *Principles of Pathobiology*, edited by R. B. Hill, Jr and M. F. La Via (New York: Oxford University Press)

Trump, B. F., Jones, R. J. and Laufer, A. (1983) *Cellular Pathobiology of Human Disease*. (New York: Gustav Fischer)

Trump, B.F. and Berezesky, I. K. (1984) Role of sodium and calcium regulation in toxic cell injury. In *Drug Metabolism and Drug Toxicity*, edited by J. R. Mitchell and M. J. Horning (New York: Raven Press)

Walter, J. B. (1982) *An Introduction to the Principles of Disease*. (Edinburgh: Churchill Livingstone)

Weissmann, G. (ed.) (1980) *Cell Biology of Inflammation*. (Amsterdam: Elsevier-North Holland)

3. Target organ pathology

All tissues and organs in the body are potential targets for the toxic effects of chemicals. In practice, effects tend to be observed more frequently in certain organs than in others and these organs will be used to illustrate the application of the principles described in Chapter 2. The same principles also apply to other organs such as the reproductive system. The commonly affected organs can be classified into three main groups:

1.   Organs or tissues associated with the route of exposure: skin, external eye, respiratory tract, gastrointestinal tract.
2.   Organs associated with metabolism and excretion: liver, kidney.
3.   Organs or tissues with selective vulnerability: nervous system, cardiovascular system and haemopoietic tissue.

The toxic responses observed in these target organs systems may be morphological, biochemical or functional derangement, or any combination of these three basic modes of response. This chapter will concentrate on the morphological aspects of target-organ toxicity and some of the direct and indirect causal mechanisms associated with this toxicity. Only non-neoplastic responses are described. These responses to chemical insult are basically the same as those following any other cause of cell injury, namely degeneration, proliferation and inflammation, but the histological appearance and diagnostic terminology may vary widely from organ to organ. However, the terminology still reflects two basic items, the location and nature of the effect.

Skin

The skin is the external covering of the body and is continuous with the lining of orifices opening onto the body surface. Its structure varies widely in different regions, from the delicate skin of the scrotum to the rough thick covering of foot-pads. It is one of the largest organs in the body and it is exposed to numerous chemicals every day. It is also the most frequently injured, and occupational skin disease accounts for a very large proportion of industrial compensation claims. Skin disease is also responsible for a lot of human misery through the psychological

51

effects of some of the more highly visible lesions. Yet, it is a sad fact that by comparison with organs such as the liver and kidney, fundamental research into cutaneous toxicology can only be described as meagre.

All surface coverings have essentially the same basic structure. There is a superficial lining of epithelial cells supported by a subepithelial connective-tissue stroma and vasculature. Most surfaces also have other specialised structures related to the particular functions of the lining membrane. In the skin, the basic components are the epidermis, dermis and adnexa (Figure 3.1). The epidermis consists largely of a dividing population of basal cells, the progeny of which slowly migrate to the surface and differentiate into the flattened keratin-rich cells of the horny layer of stratum corneum. The stratum corneum is the main protective layer of the skin. The thickness of the epidermis varies markedly in different parts of the body and in different species. The supporting tissue or dermis forms the major thickness of the skin and consists mainly of fibrous tissue and blood vessels. There are also other cells such as mast cells which may play important roles in chemical injury. The vasculature nourishing the dermis and epidermis is of major importance in the response to chemical injury. This vasculature may appear sparse relative to that in absorptive epithelia, but the phenomenon of blushing soon reveals the true extent of vascular perfusion. The hair follicles and sweat glands are the main adnexal components whose nature and extent differ markedly between species. Most mammals are hairy in comparison with man.

The two main mechanisms of skin insult are direct injury (irritation) and immune

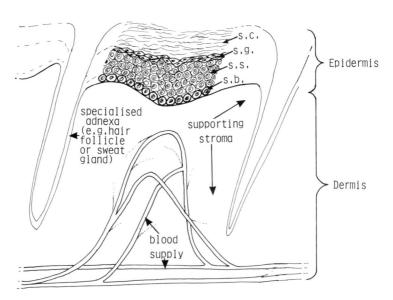

Figure 3.1. Basic organisation of the skin. s.c. = stratum corneum; s.g. = stratum granulosum; s.s. = stratum spinosum; s.b. = stratum basale.

injury (allergy). The response of the skin to these insults, like that of any other tissue is limited largely to degeneration, proliferation and inflammation or any combination of these three basic responses. The combination that is observed at any point in time depends on the nature, rate, extent, depth and duration of injury but is often dominated by the inflammatory processes. Dermatitis, variously qualified, is the most frequently used diagnosis.

Irritant dermatitis

Most adverse skin reactions to chemicals, both in industry and the general population are probably associated with irritancy. In most cases, the molecular mechanisms of injury are unknown and investigators are limited to more empirical terms such as mild or strong irritation. Unfortunately, for any one particular chemical, these terms are only valid for well-defined circumstances. For example, water may be considered non-toxic, but continued exposure to water is a major disabling factor in the military in the form of trench foot, paddy foot and related conditions. Because the effects of any one chemical is so influenced by other factors, the emphasis in this section will be on the common ranges of histological responses to direct contact injury.

In the mildest form of superficial injury, damage is restricted mainly to the epidermis. After a single (acute) injury the basal cells quickly respond to damage in the superficial layers by increasing cell division and the epidermis regenerates to normal. If the insult continues, the proliferation continues and the epidermis ultimately becomes thickened (Figure 3.2). The response to continued mild irritation is thus dominated by hyperplasia. Diagnostic terms used to define various elements of this epidermal proliferation include hyperkeratosis, hypergranulosis and acanthosis for thickening of the stratum corneum, stratum granulosum and stratum spinosum respectively. The thickened skin on the palms of a manual worker is an example of a proliferative response to low-grade continued abrasive injury. As long as the basement membrane is undamaged, mild irritation generally evokes little response in the dermis other than transient vasodilation.

The histological response to severe irritation (corrosion) begins initially as degeneration. The severity depends on the depth of penetration of the chemical, but the epidermis, basement membrane and at least the superficial dermis are killed. This evokes an inflammatory response at the junction between necrotic and viable tissue and is subsequently followed by a proliferative response of remaining epithelial and connective-tissue elements in an attempt to repair the lesion. The precursor cells for epithelial regeneration are usually derived from undamaged adnexal components such as hair follicles lying deep in the dermis. The superficiel dead layer eventually sloughs as the damage is repaired leaving a scar (Figure 3.3). Concentrated acids and alkalies are the classical strong irritants, but many organic compounds display similar attributes. Because the injury is rapid and obvious, it is relatively easy to define the causal agent involved when investigating skin lesions in man.

Normal

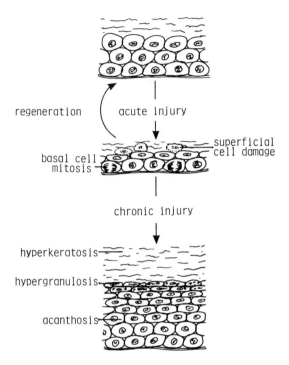

Figure 3.2. Epidermal response to mild irritation.

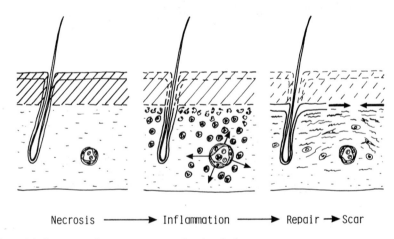

Figure 3.3. Sequence of response to corrosive chemicals.

Most forms of dermatitis fall somewhere between the two extremes of mild and severe. Continued mild to moderate injury may produce a wide range of responses including various combinations of degeneration, proliferation and inflammation, often referred to clinically as eczema. In the early stages inflammatory responses usually dominate the histological picture. Vasodilation (erythema), exudation and leucocyte emigration are prominent. Fluid may accumulate locally to form vesicles (bullae, blisters). Accumulations of polymorphs may produce microabscesses in the epidermis. Larger accumulations are known as macroabscesses or pustules. With continued irritation epithelial proliferation is increased. The skin becomes thickened and may become fissured. The differentiation of proliferating keratinocytes may be abnormal and nuclei may be retained in the horny layer. This process is known as parakeratosis. Detergents, soaps and many organic compounds can produce mild to moderate irritation following repeated or prolonged contact. However, there may be little visible response during the early stages of exposure and in clinical practice it is much more difficult to identify the cause of dermatitis than it is in patients exposed to strong irritants.

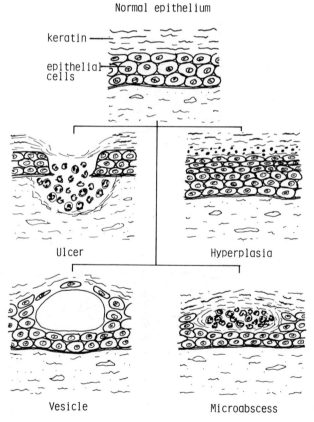

Figure 3.4. Examples of epidermal responses to moderate irritants.

In predictive toxicology, the conventional model for primary skin irritation is the rabbit. The general consensus is that the thin skin of the rabbit is generally more sensitive than that of man and is likely to err on the safe side when screening for irritants. The rabbit model is unlikely to miss comparatively strong irritants, but may be unreliable in discriminating among weak irritants. The irritation response is usually assessed by naked eye examination of exposed skin sites and scoring for changes such as oedema and erythema. Histological examination is unusual except when testing dyestuffs or other coloured substances which interfere with the assessment of erythema.

Allergic dermatitis

This is much less common than contact dermatitis due to primary irritation. Nevertheless, allergic contact dermatitis can be of great significance in industry because ordinary protective measures may be useless and affected workers may have to leave their jobs. Fortunately, most contact allergens produce sensitisation in only a small percentage of exposed persons, and of the thousands of chemicals in commercial use only a few hundred are commonly recognised as contact allergic sensitisers. However, some of these are widespread, particularly metals such as nickel and chromium, and formaldehyde is of particular concern to the toxicological pathologist.

Allergic contact dermatitis is a type IV, delayed, or cell-mediated immune reaction. Chemicals generally act as haptens, conjugating with skin proteins to form a complete antigen which elicits the immune response. If the reaction is evoked experimentally by patch testing, there is an inflammatory response at the site of contact beginning within 12 hours, reaching a peak around 24–72 hours and then slowly subsiding. Histologically, the earliest lesion is vasodilation, followed by perivascular mononuclear leucocyte cuffing. Leucocytes migrate into the epidermis which shows progressive microvesiculation and hyperplasia. In clinical practice however, the gross appearance is not unlike that of irritation. There are no distinctive clinical features that differentiate allergic contact dermatitis from irritant contact dermatitis and the basic pathologic lesion is essentially the same. This reinforces the axiom that the body's reaction to injury is limited and it is often impossible to define the causal agent on the basis of the observed response.

The guinea-pig is the usual animal model in predictive allergen testing. A variety of sensitisation and challenge protocols are in use in regulatory toxicology. Some, such as the Maximisation test, are claimed to be highly predictive in screening for potential human allergens. They are capable of detecting weak sensitisers such as the optical brighteners which produced an epidemic of allergic contact dermatitis when they were put into detergents for sale in Denmark.

Phototoxic and photoallergic dermatitis

These have essentially the same basic pathology as irritant and allergic contact dermatitis but light is a factor in their causation. Phototoxicity is the more common. It is caused by light activation of photosensitive chemicals which are present in the skin either as a result of topical application or following systemic administration. The chemicals tend to be relatively low molecular weight compounds with resonating bonds that absorb ultraviolet light. The molecular mechanisms of injury are unknown, but some reactions require oxygen suggesting possible free radical or peroxidative injury. The anthraquinone Disperse Blue, once used in bathing suits, is a classic example of topical phototoxicity, and phenothiazines, such as chlorpromazine, are well-known systemic photosensitisers. In photoallergic reactions, light facilitates conjugation of the hapten with a skin protein to form a sensitising allergen. One of the best known group of photoallergens is the halogenated salicylanilides once used as bacteriostats in soaps.

Contact urticaria

This term is used for acute wheal and flare reactions that occur within a few minutes to one hour after the skin is exposed to certain rapidly absorbable chemicals. The mechanisms are similar to these of other forms of dermatitis, namely non-immune and immune. Non-immune mechanisms seem to be the most common. The chemical has a direct influence on dermal vessel walls or indirectly causes a vascular reaction by release of vasoactive substances such as histamine and bradykinin. Certain organic acids such as cinnamic acid, benzoic acid and sorbic acid are particularly potent. Allergic contact urticuria is a Type I immune reaction mediated by IgE.

Hypopigmentation

Chemically induced depigmentation is uncommon, but can be cosmetically disastrous in non-caucasians. Skin colour is due to melanin pigments produced by melanocytes in the epidermis. Substituted phenols such as the antioxidant *p*-tertiary butyl catechol are melanocidal *in vivo* and *in vitro*. One of the best documented outbreaks is depigmentation in workers wearing rubber gloves containing the monobenzyl ether of hydroquinone. Animal models such as pigmented black guinea-pigs are adequate screens for detecting chemical depigmentation.

Acne

Acne is a lesion of the hair follicle. It results from hyperproliferation of keratinised cells in the follicle producing keratin plugs, retention of sebum and distension of the follicle lumen (comedones). If the follicle ruptures, the contents incite an inflammatory response in the surrounding dermis. Acne vulgaris is the common lesion of adolescents, but acne caused by environmental agents is termed environmental acne or acne venenata. There are many variants of environmental acne, but oil acne and chloracne are among the most important. Oil acne was once a very common occupational skin disease caused by repeated exposure to cutting oils or petroleum oils. The incidence has declined with the introduction of better hygiene. Chloracne is related to exposure to chlorinated hydrocarbons. It is more severe and persistent than ordinary oil acne. The early lesions are pale yellow cysts on the face. Histologically the first signs are thickening of the follicular epithelium followed by comedone formation. Later, the sebaceous glands disappear and the lesion becomes a keratin-filled cyst. Acnegens of current interest include polyhalogenated biphenyls (PCB, PBB) and 2,3,7,8-tetrachlorodibenzo-*p*-dioxin (TCDD). The rabbit external ear canal is the usual animal model to screen chemicals for acnegenic potential. Chemicals are applied daily for at least two weeks and histological examination is used to assess formation of hyperkeratotic masses in the follicles.

External eye

The conjunctiva, cornea and associated tissues resemble the skin in that they are directly exposed to external injury. Anatomically, the conjunctiva has a non-keratinised squamous surface epithelium supported by a vascularised stroma. The cornea also has a surface epithelium and supporting stroma, but is unique because the stroma is avascular. The main adnexal components of the external eye are various lubricating glands such as the lachrymal and Harderian glands (Figure 3.5). Injury to the eye often affects all components and terms such as keratoconjunctivitis are common. Damage may also include the internal structures of the eye such as the anterior chamber and iris. To illustrate some of the principles of injury, however, each component will be considered separately.

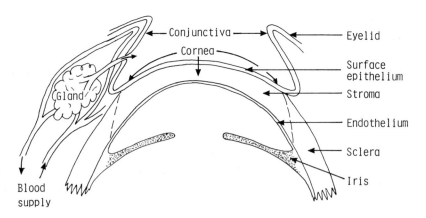

Figure 3.5. Basic organisation of the external eye.

Conjunctiva

The conjunctiva is a delicate well vascularised membrane lining the inner surface of the eyelids (palpebral conjunctiva) and the outer margin of the anterior globe (bulbar conjunctiva). The epithelium is squamous, non-keratinised with numerous mucus-secreting cells. The mechanisms and responses to injury are the same as those described in the skin. The main effect observed is inflammation (conjunctivitis) and this may be caused by direct irritation or immune injury.

Irritant conjunctivitis

Splashes of acid, solvents, detergents, strong household alkalies and the deliberate application of ophthalmic preparations may cause conjunctival injury. The injury may range from a mild short-lived conjunctivitis such as that sometimes produced by 1% solutions of ophthalmic silver nitrate, to severe injury with scarring following alkali burns.

The gross manifestations of inflammation form the basis of part of the scoring categories used in acute eye irritation studies in laboratory animals such as the Draize test. Vasodilation is scored as the category reddening, the swelling produced by fluid exudate is scored as chemosis and cellular exudates across the surface epithelium form part of the category scored as discharge. The latter also includes accumulation of secretion from mucous cells and adnexal glands. The histological appearance is typical of the various forms and stages of inflammation. Chronic inflammation and scarring are important if they lead to obstruction of the openings of the nasolachrymal duct. Tears are unable to drain away and overflow onto the skin of the face (epiphora).

Allergic conjunctivitis

Type I allergic reactions are a very common clinical condition in man, notably in hay-fever sufferers. Chemically induced IgE-mediated reactions are much less common. The usual reaction is conjunctival congestion and oedema. Many drugs used as ophthalmic preparations have also been associated with Type IV allergy. These include anaesthetics, steroids, antimicrobials and the preservatives and vehicles used in these preparations. In chronic cases, the histological appearance cannot be distinguished from other forms of chronic conjunctivitis.

Pigmentation

In man, the prolonged use of epinephrine eyedrops may result in adenochrome deposits. These deposits are pink to dark brown and have a similar appearance to particles of mascara eye liner which can also accumulate in the tarsal conjunctiva. Chronic application of preparations such as mercuric oxide or ammoniated mercury may produce mercurial deposits on the lid and conjunctiva.

Cornea

The integrity of the cornea is critical to normal vision. Transparency is associated with the rather unusual structure of the cornea. There are five major layers, a multilayered surface epithelium, Bowman's membrane, stroma, Descemet's membrane and a single-layered endothelium lining the inner surface of the cornea. The avascular stroma accounts for 90% of the thickness of the cornea in most mammals. It consists of parallel bands of collagen fibres which are about 78% hydrated. Transparency depends on this peculiar lamellar arrangement of collagen fibres and the degree of hydration. Hydration is maintained by the corneal endothelium. Chemicals may damage the surface epithelium and/or the stroma resulting in inflammatory or degenerative changes. Many of these changes are designated keratitis even though inflammatory reactions may be minimal or absent in some cases, particularly when injury is restricted to the corneal epithelium.

Epithelial responses

The surface epithelium can undergo the range of degenerative responses seen in any other tissues. These include vacuolation, pigmentation and necrosis (Figure 3.6). In man the classic example of vacuolar keratitis results from chronic exposure to n-butanol. By slit-lamp biomicroscope the vacuoles look like tiny gas bubbles in the epithelium. A more diffuse effect is cell swelling or oedema. In man this is often a delayed effect occurring several hours after exposure to certain vapours such as allyl alcohol and diisopropylamine. The effect is reversible. Epithelial pigmentation is uncommon, but has been described as an occupational hazard associated with the manufacture of hydroquinone. Hydroquinone dust reaching the eye is oxidised to benzoquinone which is brown. Accumulation of brown granules eventually produces a brown band keratopathy.

Death and loss of the corneal epithelial cells is a more serious injury, particularly if excessive. The simplest form is small areas of desquamation or erosion. This may follow splashes of neutral organic solvents in the eye, possibly because of their ability to dissolve fat in the epithelium. These small erosions can be highlighted by applying fluorescein to the cornea. Minor injuries rapidly heal by regeneration if the basement membrane is intact. Regeneration is slower in rabbits than in man. More extreme injuries will damage the underlying stroma and incite an inflammatory reaction (keratitis).

Stromal responses

The simplest response is an increase in the degree of hydration of the stroma (corneal oedema) resulting in a change in transparency of the cornea. This is visible as a cloudiness or opacity and is usually reversible. More severe stromal injuries incite an inflammatory reaction. The resultant keratitis may be classified as nonulcerative if the surface epithelium is intact or ulcerative if the epithelium is lost.

Strong acids and alkalis are notorious for producing rapid penetrating injury of the epithelium and corneal stroma. The initial reaction is oedema. The inflammatory reaction is delayed compared with that in other tissues since the cornea is avascular. Eventually, neutrophils migrate into the damaged cornea followed by an ingrowth of vessels from the vasculature at the margin (limbus) of the cornea. The ingrowth of vessels and their associated fibroblasts to repair the damaged stroma is known as pannus formation. Rabbit eyes have a rich vascular plexus at the limbus which responds rapidly and vigorously to corneal injury and pannus

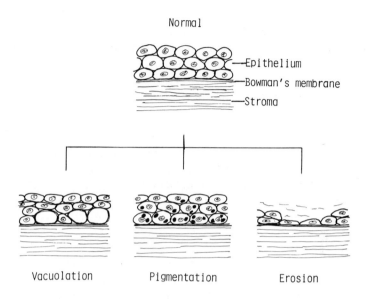

Normal

—Epithelium
—Bowman's membrane
—Stroma

Vacuolation   Pigmentation   Erosion

Figure 3.6. Corneal epithelial responses to injury.

formation occurs more readily than in humans. It usually occurs 4–7 days after injury and following diffuse injury will envelop the whole cornea within two weeks. The pannus may eventually regress, but does not disappear entirely. In man, pannus formation is usually associated with chronic disease and is not an acute irritative effect. It also tends to disappear following healing of the cornea.

The corneal damage caused by acids and alkalis is related to the pH and in the case of acids to the nature of the cation. Mineral acids such as hydrochloric acid cause little injury unless the pH is less than 2.5. Organic acids such as picric, tungstic and tannic acid may produce lesions even when buffered. Acid burns vary in severity from those that heal completely to those causing perforation of the globe. The reaction seen in the first few hours is a reasonable measure of the long term damage to be expected. Alkali burns are more common in man because of the widespread use of chemicals such as sodium hydroxide and ammonia. The effect of caustic injury is delayed compared with that of acid burns and the nature of the cation has very little bearing on the ultimate severity of the burn. The pH, concentration and duration of exposure are the critical factors. In general, the pH of solutions causing opacities is usually greater than 11.

Iris

This is an internal structure of the globe, but there are close anatomic relationships of both nerves and blood vessels between the cornea and the iris. In addition, the aqueous humour bathes both the iris and posterior surface of the cornea.

Some irritants, such as ammonia, penetrate the cornea rapidly and appear within the aqueous humour within a few seconds. It is not surprising therefore that topically applied chemicals may affect the aqueous humour and iris, and that evaluations of these ocular components are routinely included in eye irritation studies.

The iris is a highly vascular structure and most reactions to irritants begin with vasodilation (hyperaemia) and swelling due to oedema. With severe irritation, proteinaceous and cellular exudate may spill over into the fluid of the anterior chamber and alter the refractive index of the aqueous fluid to produce what is known as an aqueous flare when a beam of light passes through the globe. If the inflammation is of the haemorrhagic type, the accumulation of free blood in the anterior chamber is known as hyphema. In suppurative inflammation, the accumulation of pus is termed hypopyon. The inflammation (iritis) may resolve, but in severe cases fibrous repair may produce adhesions between the iris and posterior aspect of the cornea or the anterior part of the lens capsule. The adhesions are termed synechiae and may interfere with flow and drainage of the aqueous humour and cause a painful swelling of the globe known as glaucoma. This is another example of the way post-inflammatory fibrous repair can have disastrous sequelae if it occurs in critical locations.

Respiratory tract

Breathing is an involuntary activity, during which the respiratory tract is exposed to chemicals in the inspired air and is at risk to toxic injury. The causal mechanisms and responses to injury are essentially the same as in other tissues, but are complicated by several factors. The two main factors are the physicochemical nature of the agent and the gross functional anatomy of the respiratory tract. These have a marked effect on the location and nature of tissue injury. These two factors are often interdependent, but they will be described briefly as separate entities to introduce the principles of respiratory tract toxicology.

The gross functional anatomy of the respiratory system is a major determinant of the site of deposition of inhaled substances. The respiratory system has two main components: a conducting system, designed to process, deliver and remove air; and a gaseous exchange system by which blood is oxygenated and decarbonated. The latter, the respiratory acinus, is relatively simple consisting mainly of alveoli. The conducting system, on the other hand, is fairly complex because it also performs other functions such as olfaction and vocalisation. It is conventionally divided into the nasopharynx and tracheobronchiolar tree or alternatively described as the upper and lower airways (Figure 3.7). At a more basic level the respiratory tract can be reduced to a conducting system of decreasing diameter, but increasing volume and surface area that leads into a massive area for gaseous exchange. As described below this physical structure has a marked influence on the site of deposition of airborne toxins, especially particles.

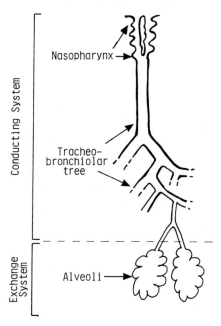

Figure 3.7. Gross anatomy of the respiratory system.

The second important factor in respiratory tract toxicology is the physico-chemical nature of the material. Inhaled substances may exist in various physical forms, namely gas, vapour, and liquid or solid aerosols. A gas is a substance, the physical state of which is without fixed volume; a vapour is a gaseous form of a substance which is normally liquid; an aerosol is a collection of fine particles either liquid or solid, which are dispersed in a gas; a mist is a fine liquid aerosol; and a fume is a fine solid aerosol. The main physical factors affecting the site of deposition of these various forms of chemical are size and water solubility. Large particles in the range 5–30 μm aerodynamic diameter will tend to be trapped by impaction as air flows turbulently through the convoluted channels of the nasopharyngeal region. Smaller particles 1–5 μm diameter may enter the smaller airways of the tracheobronchiolar tree and tend either to impact as these airways branch or to sediment as airflow slows before reaching the respiratory acinus. Only the very small particles 1 μm or less in aerodynamic diameter such as in fumes are likely to diffuse into the alveolar region in large quantities. Gases and vapours on the other hand may diffuse throughout the respiratory tree and water solubility is usually the major determining factor of their site of action. Highly water soluble substances such as SO_2 and other anhydrous acid vapours will rapidly dissolve in the aqueous phases of the upper airways and little will remain in the inspired air conducted to the deeper levels of the lung. Relatively insoluble gases such as O_3 will not dissolve so readily and may diffuse to the smaller airways and alveoli in sufficient quantities to cause damage.

The nature of the observed response to injury is to some extent conditioned by the histological organisation of the respiratory tract at the site of chemical deposition. The surface epithelium becomes simpler and flatter from the external nares to the alveolus. Similarly, the supporting stroma with its adnexae diminish until at the alveolar level it consists mainly of blood vessels (Figure 3.8). Because the type of epithelium, nature and amount of stroma and adnexa, and the degree of vascularity vary at different levels in the respiratory tract, the sensitivity to injury and the nature of the pathological response may appear very variable. To illustrate the variability in observed effects, and some of the causal mechanisms producing these effects, the principles of respiratory tract pathology will be illustrated using the two primary sites of disease, the conducting airways and the alveoli.

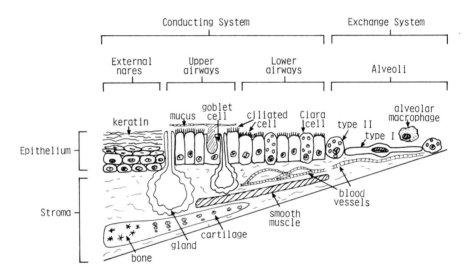

Figure 3.8. Basic organisation of the respiratory tract.

Conducting airways

The conducting airways extend from the external nares to the terminal bronchioles. The two main mechanisms of injury to the epithelium and associated tissues by airborne chemicals are direct injury and immune injury and the responses the same as those in other tissues, namely degeneration, proliferation and inflammation. The latter often dominates the histological picture and as in the skin the most frequent diagnoses are various forms of '-itis'.

Irritant airway disease

The response to inhaled irritants depends on the potency of the chemical, concentration, and the extent and duration of exposure. In most cases the molecular mechanisms of injury are unknown and the toxicologist can only describe the responses. Mild damage is restricted mainly to the epithelial layers. Most of the epithelium in the conducting airways consists of a mixture of ciliated cells, non-ciliated cells and secretory cells. In the upper airways goblet cells are the main secretory component whereas Clara cells predominate at the bronchiolar level. The ciliated cells are the most vulnerable to damage. The most frequent degenerative changes in these cells are loss of cilia, necrosis and sloughing of cells into the airway lumen. Necrosis and desquamation of non-ciliated and secretory cells are less frequently observed. After acute mild insult the non-ciliated cells proliferate and the epithelium regenerates to normal. In the tracheobronchial tree, non-ciliated basal cells are the main proliferating population. In the bronchioles, the Clara cell is the main precursor cell for regeneration. Because of the delicate nature of the respiratory tract epithelium and the close proximity of subepithelial blood vessels, an inflammatory response occurs to all but the mildest form of injury. Many lesions are therefore diagnosed as inflammations such as rhinitis, tracheitis and bronchiolitis and qualified as acute, subacute and chronic depending on the stage of the response. The site of injury depends largely on the physical properties of the irritant, but in most cases changes are most prominent in the upper airways.

If the insult persists, the hyperplasia continues and leads to an abnormal epithelium (Figure 3.9). This may consist of one or more of the following types, undifferentiated basal cells (hyperplasia), squamous cells (squamous metaplasia) and goblet cells (goblet cell metaplasia). This sort of injury is produced by chronic exposure to irritants such as SO_2, NO_2, O_3 HCHO and tobacco smoke. Ultimately, dysplasia and neoplasia may develop as a result of long-term exposure. Examples include nasal tumours in formaldehyde-exposed rats and lung cancer in tobacco smokers.

With severe irritants, such as high concentrations of toluene diisocyanate, most of the epithelium is destroyed together with the underlying stroma. If the animal survives, fibrosis is a major component of the repair process producing distortion and dysfunction of the conducting airways. In practice, many irritants produce responses intermediate between mild and severe and various combinations of degeneration, inflammation and proliferation may be observed. Because these responses to chemical injury are non-specific, it is essential to use animal models free of upper respiratory tract infections in inhalation toxicology. Unfortunately, this is not always possible because viral infections such as Sendai are endemic in many colonies.

Asthma

The contraction of airway smooth muscle causes a respiratory difficulty known as bronchial asthma. Asthma may be caused by at least three mechanisms, allergy, irritation and a disturbance in the control of pharmacologic mediator release. Allergic bronchial asthma has been associated with a number of agents including

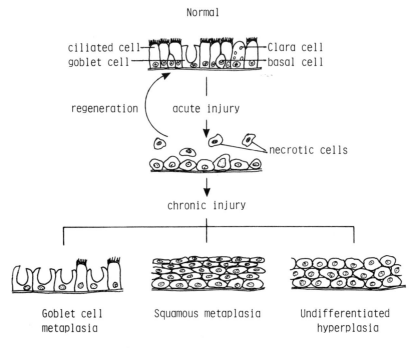

Figure 3.9. Airway epithelial response to mild acute and chronic injury.

animal proteins, plant and bacterial enzymes, certain platinum salts and a variety of chemicals used in the plastics industry. This may be relatively difficult to produce in animal models and much of our toxicological experience comes from studies in man. Clinical experience with a wide variety of chemicals suggests that Type I and III immune reactions may occur in the conducting airways. Type I reactions to organic dusts are relatively common in everyday life as any hay fever sufferer must know, but organic dusts are also an important cause of occupational disease. IgE-mediated histamine release produces an immediate onset reaction. In the nose, rhinitis is the characteristic symptom, but in lower airways histamine and other mediators cause smooth muscle contraction resulting in bronchospasm. The histological picture in the airways is vasodilation, oedema, increased mucous secretion and eosinophil infiltration. Type III immune reactions occur in response to some materials, often organic dusts, but these are more difficult to study and often overlap with alveolar disease. Type III allergic respiratory bronchiolitis may play a role in a second form of asthma which has a delayed onset compared with the more frequently encountered immediate-onset disease.

Irritant asthma may result from exposure to many gases and fumes such as sulphur dioxide, formaldehyde and various household and cosmetic sprays. The responses are thought to be mediated primarily through vagal reflex pathways resulting in acetylcholine release and smooth-muscle contraction. Contraction may also result from direct pharmacologic activity of environmental agents such as the adrenergic partial agonist activity of certain diisocyanates and possibly trimellitic anhydride. A pharmacologically-induced bronchoconstriction probably occurs in the occupational disease known as byssinosis. Deposition of inhaled cotton fibres induces the liberation of mediators such as SRS-A and histamine.

Sensory irritation

This is the nasopharyngeal equivalent to irritant bronchial asthma. Stimulation of the trigeminal nerve endings in the nasal mucosa of mice by airborne irritants leads to a reflex decrease in respiratory rate. This phenomenon has been used as a model for predicting the potential of a chemical to cause sensory irritation of the eyes, nose and throat in man.

Systemic airway injury

The conducting airways may be injured by systemically administered chemicals. One of the best studied cytotoxic chemicals is 4-ipomeanol. This is a naturally occurring furan derivative found in moldy sweet potatoes and thought to be responsible for pulmonary disease in cattle with access to potatoes in their diet. In rodent models, the characteristic lesion is necrosis of the bronchiolar Clara cells. These are an important site of cytochrome P-450 mono-oxygenase activity in the lung and 4-ipomeanol toxicity is probably due to the *in vivo* formation of a chemically reactive metabolite capable of alkylating tissue macromolecules. Bronchospasm and asthma may also be produced by systemic chemicals. The acute Type I allergic penicillin reaction is the prototype. Intolerance to oral acetylsalicylic acid is also associated with bronchospasm, but the pathogenesis is unknown.

Alveoli

The alveoli are lined by two main types of epithelial cells (Figure 3.10). Type I cells (squamous pneumonocytes) have flattened nuclei and thin, but very extensive cytoplasm covering most of the alveolar wall. Because the cell has few organelles and a very large surface area it is very susceptible to injury. The basement membrane supporting the Type I cells is closely apposed or fused with that of the underlying capillary endothelial cells. The latter are the predominant cell type in the alveolar wall. It is convenient to treat the epithelial–endothelial complex as a unit both in terms of its function in gaseous exchange and in the pathological changes caused by injury. Type II cells (granular pneumonocytes) are disposed throughout the alveoli between Type I cells. Although they are more numerous than the Type I cell, they are cuboidal in shape and occupy far less of the alveolar surface area. The prime function of this cell is the production of pulmonary surfactant and it is generally more resistant to injury than the Type

I cell. The other main cell type is the alveolar macrophage which plays an important role in removing particulates from the alveoli. Phagocytosis of toxic particulates may injure macrophages and ultimately cause alveolar damage. This is described in the section on pneumoconiosis. Stromal cells such as fibroblasts are infrequent, but may increase sufficiently during chronic inflammatory reactions to interfere with gaseous exchange and compromise lung function.

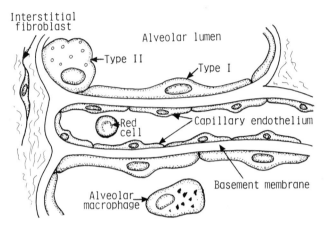

Figure 3.10. Basic organisation of the alveolus.

Irritant alveolitis

Most direct toxins entering the alveoli primarily affect Type I cells and their associated endothelial cells. Following acute injury the epithelium and/or endothelial cells may swell, disrupt, distort or lose their connections with others, leaving large areas of basement membrane uncovered. This allows fluid to move into the alveolar lumen from the capillaries and oedema or serofibrinous and then cellular exudate is the dominant histological response to cell injury. The inflammatory response obscures the earlier degenerative changes in the epithelial and endothelial cells. This early phase of alveolar damage is often referred to as acute alveolitis to emphasise the prominence of the acute exudative phase of inflammation.

The sequel to acute injury depends as in all tissues on the potency and concentration of the toxic agent and duration of exposure (Figure 3.11). Potent diffusing toxins produce a severe vascular reaction and cause diffuse septal and alveolar flooding. The fluid prevents gaseous exchange and the animal dies before any further pathological changes develop. Following acute mild non-lethal damage, excess fluid is removed and the resistant Type II cells proliferate and re-line the alveoli. The cells subsequently differentiate into Type I cells. Complete regeneration to normal can be effected by differentiation of Type II cells into Type I epithelium.

If the chemical is moderately irritant and causes significant damage to the basement membrane and stroma as well as to the epithelial cells this incites fibroblastic repair and septal fibrous scarring results. This fibrotic reaction may extend into the alveolar lumen if serofibrinous exudate is incompletely removed producing even further alveolar distortion. These fibrotic alveoli are generally lined by atypical Type II cells. The lining of alveoli by Type II cells either in the early phases of repair following mild damage or as an endstage of more severe damage is often referred to as alveolar epithelialisation or cuboidal metaplasia. Occasionally the alveoli may be re-lined by a proliferation of bronchiolar epithelium. This is termed alveolar bronchiolisation; or if extensive or distorted to produce a tumour-like condition, the term adenomatosis is sometimes used. If low grade irritation persists, the characteristic features of chronic inflammation are hyperplasia of Type II cells accompanied by fibrous and lymphocytic thickening of the interstitium. Intra-alveolar accumulation of macrophages may also be a prominent feature.

Alternative diagnoses for acute and chronic alveolitis are acute and chronic interstitial pneumonitis or pneumonia. The term interstitial is a commonly used qualifier of inflammatory reactions. It refers to a reaction dominated by a response such as leucocyte infiltration or fibrosis in the stroma supporting a functional epithelium. For example, a marked inflammatory reaction in the stroma supporting kidney tubular epithelium may be diagnosed as interstitial nephritis to emphasise the stromal inflammatory response. In the same way, the major cellular reaction in many alveolar injuries is in the supporting septum justifying the use of interstitial as a qualifying term.

In many cases, the molecular mechanisms of chemical injury to the alveolus are unknown and non-specific terms such as irritation are used. In other cases, the proposed mechanisms fall into the main general groups of direct cytotoxicity described in Chapter 2. Phosgene, for example, is hydrolysed in the respiratory tract to carbon dioxide and hydrochloric acid. The nascent hydrogen chloride directly damages the alveolar lining cells resulting in alveolar oedema. Ozone, high concentrations of oxygen and various oxides such as nitrogen dioxide possibly act through lipid peroxidation of cell membranes. The covalent binding of oxygenated intermediates is a possible mechanism in the production of pulmonary oedema by perchloroethylene.

Allergic alveolitis

Reactions to inhaled organic dusts are the most frequent form of immune alveolar injury in man. This is usually referred to as hypersensitivity pneumonitis or extrinsic allergic alveolitis. The classic prototype is 'farmer's lung' caused by the spores of moulds growing on warm damp hay. Equivalent diseases have been described in mushroom pickers, sugar cane workers, cork manufacturers and in several other occupations. High levels of precipitating antibody are usually present in the blood and acute attacks usually develop 5–6 hours after exposure. This is consistent with a Type III immune reaction. In chronic disease, there are features of both Type III and Type IV allergic reactions. The disease is difficult to reproduce in animal models.

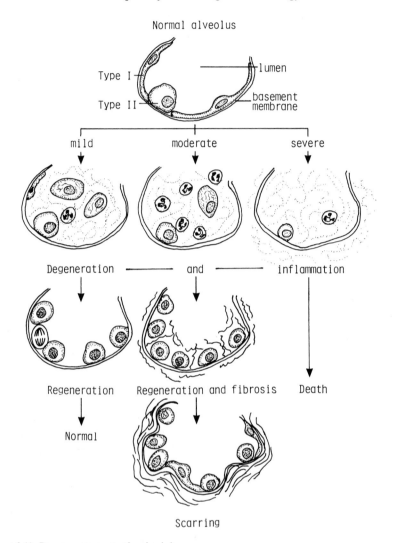

Figure 3.11. Response to acute alveolar injury.

Pneumoconiosis

This is the deposition of inorganic dust in the lung and the tissue's reaction to its presence (Figure 3.12). Most dust is deposited in the conducting airways, trapped by mucus and removed on the 'mucociliary escalator'. Soluble dusts deposited in alveoli may be cleared by dissolution, but insoluble particles are primarily removed by the alveolar macrophage. The severity of pneumoconiosis is primarily related to the toxicity of dust to the alveolar macrophage. Alveolar macrophages originate from bone marrow-derived, circulating monocytes which migrate into alveolar lumen. They differentiate into large aerobic cells dependent on oxidative phosphorylation and a relatively high oxygen tension which is consistent with the unique microenvironment in which they reside. In contrast to the neutrophil, they cannot metabolise or phagocytose effectively in a hypoxic liquid environment. They are also distinct from the peritoneal macrophages which are sometimes used as models for predicting toxic effects of chemicals on macrophages.

The toxicity of dusts to the alveolar macrophage varies widely. Most dusts are relatively non-toxic and after phagocytosing the particles the macrophage clears the alveoli by migrating on to the mucociliary escalator or into the interstitium and then via lymphatics to the regional lymph nodes. With heavy dust burdens, such as in coal worker's anthracosis, macrophages cannot keep pace with dust intake and particle-laden cells form focal accumulations in the alveoli adjacent to small bronchioles. This dust is relatively non-toxic and cell aggregates (dust cell nests) may remain viable for a considerable time. When cells die they incite little or no fibrosis and remain as non-progressive focal aggregates termed macules. Some dusts, however, are toxic to alveolar macrophages. The most significant are the crystalline forms of silica (SiO_2) such as quartz, and asbestos.

Silicosis is an occupational disease in people exposed to a high concentration of silica dust over a period of years. It is characterised by progressive pulmonary fibrosis, but the exact causal mechanisms have not been defined. Cytotoxic and immunological mechanisms are the most frequently quoted hypotheses. Most research has centred around cytotoxic effects on the alveolar macrophage. Ingested silica appears to injure the lysosome and cause release of fibrogenic factors leading to collagen synthesis and fibrosis. The typical end result is fibrotic nodules consisting of concentric bundles of collagen which frequently have a hypocellular or hyaline appearance. Simple fibrotic nodules are of relatively little functional significance, but they may fuse or progress to produce a disabling massive fibrosis.

Asbestos is a generic name for a group of fibrous silicates. Many of these are fibrogenic, but the relative potency and mechanisms of toxicity are still in some doubt. Although the fibres are cytotoxic to macrophages *in vitro*, the correlation with *in vivo* fibrogenicity is low. The physical properties of the fibre appear to be more significant and long fibres ($>20 \mu$m) are more fibrogenic than shorter ones. These may be too large for complete phagocytosis by the cell and partly ingested fibres would provide ample opportunity for enzyme leakage and subsequent tissue damage. The tissue reaction in human lungs is variable. The term asbestosis is generally reserved for an interstitial fibrosis which usually begins at the periphery of the lower lobe and progressively destroys the respiratory tissue. Other responses are focal fibrous plaques on the parietal pleura and diaphragm, and sometimes a tumour of the pleura termed mesothelioma.

Phospholipidosis

This refers to accumulation of surfactant material in the alveoli. The rat seems

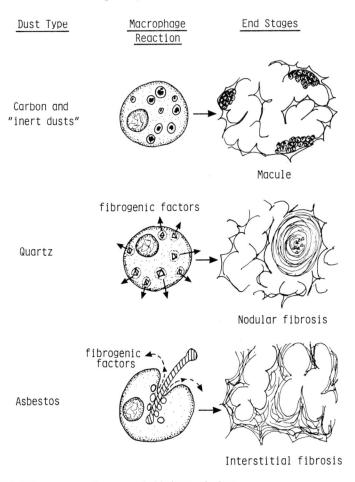

Figure 3.12. Pulmonary reaction to respirable inorganic dusts.

more prone to develop this condition than many other species. The production and catabolism of alveolar surfactant is incompletely understood. In general terms it is produced by the Type II cells and catabolised at least in part by alveolar macrophages which either transport it to the mucociliary escalator or degrade it via phospholipases. Material will accumulate because of either excess production or decreased catabolism. Certain dusts, notably quartz, may stimulate phospholipid production and secretion by Type II cells following acute high level exposure. Alveolar macrophages take up this material, and if removal is overwhelmed by excess production they appear histologically as large vacuolated cells (foam cells) in the alveolar lumen. Phospholipidosis may also be induced by systemically administered chemicals such as chlorphentermine, chlorcyclizine, amitryptiline and chloroquine. The mechanisms are unclear. However, a common feature of phospholipidosis-inducing drugs is their amphiphilic structure suggesting that they may attach to phospholipids and inhibit their catabolism by alveolar macrophages.

Emphysema

Unless otherwise qualified, emphysema means abnormal enlargement of airspaces distal to the terminal bronchiole accompanied by destructive changes in the alveolar walls (Figure 3.13). In man, it is usually associated with low level, chronic exposure to toxic inhalants continued for many years. Cigarette smoking is the major cause. Cigarette smoke and most of the important occupational inhalants are complex mixtures and the molecular mechanisms of emphysema production are largely unknown. It is also difficult to produce experimentally in animals exposed to respiratory irritants. In these experiments infusion of fixative into the lung is a common necropsy practice and care must be taken to avoid an emphysema-like artefact caused by overdistending the lungs. One current

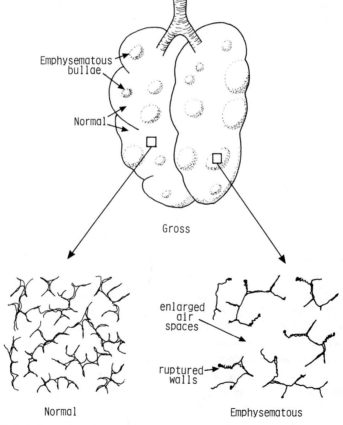

Figure 3.13. Pathology of emphysema.

hypothesis is that emphysema results from enzymatic lysis of alveolar connective tissue fibres, particularly elastin. This is followed by breakdown of alveolar walls under the mechanical stresses associated with normal or forced respiration. This elastolysis theory is supported experimentally in the production of emphysema by intratracheal administration of proteolytic enzymes such as papain, by the demonstration of elastases in neutrophils and macrophages and by the association of emphysema with genetically determined deficiency of serum protease inhibitors such as α-1-antitrypsin. However, despite this circumstantial evidence there is no conclusive proof of increased connective-tissue breakdown in emphysema in man.

Systemic alveolar injury

The alveoli are also susceptible to injury by chemicals in the circulating blood. These may be cytotoxic reactions, as in the case of paraquat and bleomycin, or Type III allergic reactions such as those occasionally associated with sulphonamide, penicillin and nitrofurantoin therapy. Because of the close epithelial–endothelial relationship in the alveolar wall, the pathological changes are essentially the same as those following inhaled toxins namely exudative, proliferative and fibrosing alveolitis in their various forms and combinations.

Gastrointestinal tract

Chemicals may be introduced into the gastrointestinal tract either deliberately in the form of drugs or alcohol, or involuntarily as pesticide residues or additives in the food we eat. The risk of gastrointestinal injury is therefore quite high. With medicines in particular, side effects are fairly common in man. Similarly, the oral route of chemical administration is the one most frequently used in toxicity studies in animals and gastrointestinal injury is common.

In most cases, the mechanism of injury is direct irritation, and as in other tissues, the response is degeneration, inflammation or proliferation depending on the nature and extent of exposure and the site of injury. The latter is important because the structure of the gastrointestinal mucosa is not uniform throughout its length (Figure 3.14). The initial part is lined by stratified squamous epithelium similar to that of skin. In man, this terminates at the oesophagus, but in many animals continues into the stomach, for example as the forestomach of rat or rumen of sheep. The true glandular stomach has an epithelium thrown into folds or crypts. In the fundic region there are three specialised cell types in the epithelium, secreting mucus, acid and enzymes respectively. In the pyloric region, mucus-secreting elements dominate. The epithelium of the small intestine is thrown into finger-like folds or villi. These decrease in size along the length of the small intestine, and as the large intestine arises, the epithelium becomes organised into crypt-like structures similar to those in the stomach. Finally, the epithelium becomes stratified squamous again near the anus. This section will briefly review some of the pathological responses produced by chemicals in these major regions of the gastrointestinal tract.

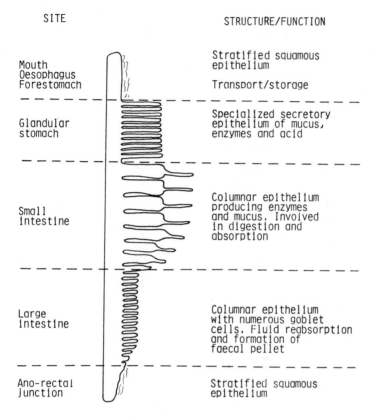

Figure 3.14. Basic organisation of the gastrointestinal tract.

Forestomach

The forestomach is a common site of irritation, particularly in the rat which is one of the primary species used in toxicology. The response to injury is essentially similar to that seen in the skin. Mild injury produces minor proliferative changes resulting in hyperkeratosis or acanthosis. Stronger irritants cause necrosis of the epithelium and incite a pronounced inflammatory reaction in the underlying stroma (Figure 3.15). If injury persists, a marked regenerative proliferation may occur resulting in a thickened epithelium thrown into wart-like configurations easily visible at necropsy. With certain chemicals this papillomatous hyperplasia may give rise to neoplasms.

Glandular stomach

In principle, the specialised epithelium of the glandular stomach should be more

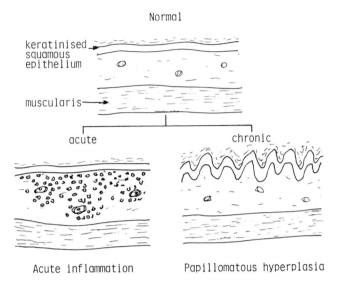

Figure 3.15. Response of rat forestomach to acute and chronic irritation.

susceptible to irritation than the stratified squamous keratinised epithelium of the forestomach. It is, however, protected by a mucous layer and irritation is less frequent than might be expected. Some chemicals though, such as non-steroidal anti-inflammatory agents (NSAIs), are notorious for producing gastric injury even at therapeutic doses, and this is one of the main side effects of this class of drugs.

The mechanism by which NSAIs and other gastric irritants such as detergents injure the mucosa is not fully understood. Impairment of the gastric mucosal barrier plays an important role. The barrier impedes diffusion of acid from the lumen into the mucosa and impedes diffusion of Na^+ from the mucosal interstitial space into the lumen. The exact nature and location of the barrier is not known, but mucus and the plasma membrane of the surface epithelial cells must play a major role. Artificial detergents and natural detergents such as bile salts may disrupt the barrier by disturbing the mucus gel and the arrangement of lipid membranes. Other lipid-soluble substances may penetrate the barrier and injure the cells maintaining the barrier. Ethanol and organic acids are in this category. Back diffusion of acid into the mucosa may enhance cytotoxicity and also release histamine from the mucosal stores to produce a variety of pathophysiological effects. In the case of NSAIs other mechanisms are also operative since these damage the stomach following systemic administration. They probably compromise the protective role of mucosal prostaglandins. The main reaction to NSAIs and other irritants is either focal damage such as erosions and ulcers, or a diffuse gastritis (Figure 3.16).

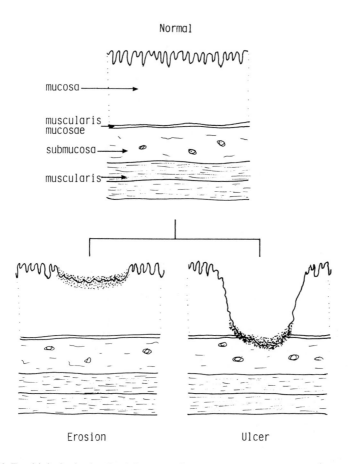

Figure 3.16. Focal injuries in the glandular stomach.

Erosion

An erosion is focal necrosis of the epithelium and associated stroma restricted to the superficial layers of the glandular mucosa. They are usually multiple and frequently occur at the tips of the folds in the stomach lining. In the early stage, there is haemorrhage from the damaged area and at necropsy this may appear as brown threads or plugs emanating from the mucosal injury. Inflammation and repair follow, and in the absence of repeated insult the mucosa will return to normal. In some cases, the mucosa may return to normal despite repeated insult, a process termed adaptive cytoprotection. This has important consequences for the assessment of chemicals for gastric irritation. Chemicals may irritate the stomach lining in the first few days of a toxicity study, but if the stomach is only examined after several days of chemical administration there may be no apparent effect. Adaptive cytoprotection to a mild irritant may also make the mucosa refractory to injury by much stronger irritants. Protection is probably associated with an increased synthesis of prostaglandins in the mucosa.

Ulcer

Ulcers are deeper injuries to the stomach lining and are often solitary or few in number. They extend beyond the mucosa into the underlying tissues and in some cases may extend through the muscular wall of the stomach and open into the abdominal cavity. The latter are termed perforating ulcers. Ulceration incites a more pronounced inflammatory reaction than erosion and healing is by regeneration and fibrosis. The regenerated epithelium may be different from that normally present and resemble intestinal epithelium or the mucus-secreting epithelium of the pylorus. These are forms of metaplasia. Fibrous scars in the pyloric region may compromise the pyloric sphincter and interfere with gastric emptying.

Diffuse gastritis

Some chemicals produce a more diffuse irritation of the stomach mucosa. The acute forms of diffuse gastritis range from a mild superficial injury, such as that produced by aspirin or spiced foods in man, to a deep necrotising gastritis that follows the ingestion of caustic materials. More chronic forms of mild irritation may result in hyperplasia of the gastric mucosa. This is seen, for example, in rats and pigs fed sulphite-rich diets.

Small intestine

The small intestine is one of the largest organs in the body in terms of surface area. It is also one of the body's most rapidly dividing tissues. Functionally it is concerned with transport of fluid and nutrients and to a lesser extent with xenobiotic metabolism. These processes are interlinked with metabolic processes occurring in the lumen of the bowel associated with digestive enzymes and the gut microflora. It is this complex physiological balance that is most likely to be deranged by chemicals. This may result in functional disturbances such as fluid and electrolyte loss, malabsorption, vomiting and diarrhoea. Morphological effects are less frequently encountered (Figure 3.17).

Erosion and ulcer

The mucosa of the small intestine is covered by a single layer of columnar epithelium and theoretically is as susceptible to erosion or ulceration as the gastric mucosa. However, ulceration is less frequently encountered. The reasons for this include a reduced concentration of chemical following gastric absorption, dilution of the chemical by gastric and intestinal fluids, dispersion over a larger surface area, a more rapid transit and a change in pH of the intestinal fluids. Enterohepatic recirculation may alter this situation. For example, in the dog, many NSAIs are excreted predominantly in the bile and undergo a pronounced enterohepatic recirculation leading to prolonged exposure of the mucosa to potential irritants. This accounts at least in part for the relative sensitivity of the dog gastrointestinal tract to this class of chemicals. The pathology of these ulcers is similar to that in the stomach ranging from superficial to perforating, depending on the depth of the injury. A more diffuse irritation and inflammation may occur if caustic substances or metals such as arsenic and mercury enter the intestine. This diffuse inflammation of the bowel is known as enteritis.

Villous stunting

The long slender villi of the small intestine may become stunted by chemicals that inhibit division of the rapidly dividing precursor cells in the crypts at the base of the villus. Methotrexate, for example, inhibits DNA synthesis via its effect on dihydrofolate reductase. It causes an acute injury to the intestinal epithelium characterised by reduced mitoses in the crypts and shortened villi. Stunting may also occur if chemicals cause loss or desquamation of the apical absorptive cells faster than they can be replaced by cell division in the crypts. In this case the crypts will elongate as a result of increased cell division, but the villi will be shorter and the villus : crypt ratio alters. Chronic ingestion of ethanol or iodoacetamide can produce this type of effect in rats. Finally, villous atrophy can also be produced via immune mechanisms. Coeliac disease in man is associated with a sensitivity to gluten, a protein from wheat. The underlying abnormality appears to be an abnormal immune response to gluten and is followed by a diffuse villous atrophy in the jejunum. The mucosa returns to normal if gluten is removed from the diet.

Lipid accumulation

Chemicals occasionally produce other effects on the intestinal mucosa, such as lipid accumulations. Tetracyclines, for example, may cause fatty change in the epithelial cells, an effect consistent with their effect on the liver. Other lipoidal chemicals such as erythromycin esters and detergent-like materials may permeate the absorptive epithelium and be phagocytosed by macrophages in the underlying stroma. They interfere with lysosomal digestion and accumulate in the macrophage to produce clusters of foam cells in the lamina propria of the villus. With continued ingestion, foam cells may appear in other tissues such as the mesenteric lymph node or liver.

Diarrhoea

This is a common response to ingested chemicals. In some cases it is associated with obvious mucosal injury such as enteritis. In other cases there may be little or no evidence of mucosal damage. In these instances, the effect may be due to sensory irritation, to a direct effect on the muscle cells, to hyperosmolarity of the chemical in the bowel lumen or to an effect on the enterocyte membranes controlling fluid and electrolyte transport. Detergents in the diet, for example, may exfoliate or release the brush border membrane of the small intestinal villi resulting in malabsorption of nutrients and water, causing diarrhoea.

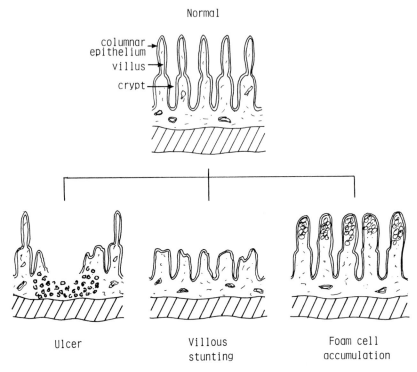

Figure 3.17. Examples of intestinal lesions.

Large intestine

The mechanisms and responses to injury in the large bowel are essentially similar to those in the stomach and small intestine. NSAIs and other chemicals may produce erosions and ulcers or a more widespread inflammation such as caecitis (typhlitis) or colitis. Chronic ingestion of certain chemicals may produce mucosal hyperplasia, squamous metaplasia or occasionally lead to neoplasia. Other chemicals may accumulate. For example, high doses of certain types of carrageenin, which are polysaccharides extracted from seaweed, may accumulate in histiocytes in the wall of the large bowel of rats and eventually lead to mucosal ulceration.

Some dietary substances may have osmotic effects and in rats, for example, may cause gross enlargement of the caecum. Raw or chemically modified starches fed as the sole or major carbohydrate constituent of diet can produce caecal enlargement to such an extent that respiration is impaired and the rat may die. The size of the rat caecum is controlled by the osmotic value of the caecal contents and caecal enlargement following administration of starches and related substances is a process of physiological adaptation. It is rapidly reversible if the animals are returned to a normal diet.

Finally, chemicals may have indirect effects if they modify the intestinal flora. Antibiotics are the prime example of this group. In rats, caecal enlargement is a frequent response to antibiotic administration, but the effect is generally less severe than that produced by starches. In other species antibiotics may suppress the normal flora and allow an overgrowth of toxin-producing bacteria such as *Clostridium difficile* or allow fungal growth and invasion of the mucosa to produce ulcers.

Liver

The hepatobiliary system consists of the liver, gall bladder (except in rat) and the extrahepatic bile duct. Chemical effects on the gall bladder and extrahepatic bile duct are uncommon. However, the liver is a common target organ in toxicity studies in animals and to a lesser extent in humans deliberately or accidentally exposed to chemicals. There are three main reasons for the vulnerability of the liver. Many chemicals are taken orally and the liver is the first organ to be exposed to chemicals absorbed into the hepatic portal vein from the gastrointestinal tract. During this exposure the liver may remove (clear) most or all of the chemical from the blood and is often exposed to higher concentrations of potential toxins than any other organ in the body. Secondly, the liver is the major site of biotransformation and may generate toxic metabolites from chemicals taken into the liver cell. Finally, biliary excretion is a major route of elimination of xenobiotics, and chemicals or their metabolites concentrated during this process may reach toxic levels.

There are various ways to classify hepatotoxicity, but most classifications are based on either causal mechanisms or type of effect. Research into hepatotoxicity has been the foundation of much of our current knowledge and thinking on the causal mechanisms of tissue injury. However, the gaps are still too great to classify injury much further than simple concepts such as predictable dose-dependent injury associated with potent hepatotoxins such as CCl_4, and injury that is unpredictable or idiosyncratic due to some unusual feature in the host, such as aberrant metabolic pathways or hypersensitivity. Hepatotoxicity will therefore be approached initially from the traditional standpoint of morphological effects based on the location and nature of response followed by a discussion of some of the causal mechanisms.

The liver is composed of lobules and location of injury is often specified morphologically in terms of its position within the lobule. Unfortunately, there are two definitions of lobule, the classic hexagonal lobule of the anatomist and the functional liver acinus (Figure 3.18). In the classic lobule, the anatomical relationship between the hepatocyte, vascular supply and biliary tree is considered to form a hexagon. The portal triads of hepatic portal vein, hepatic artery and bile duct are at the corners and the terminal hepatic venule (central vein) forms an axis in the middle. The concept of periportal, midzonal and centrilobular injury is based on this type of lobule. Although such a lobule can be visualised anatomically in species like the pig, other studies suggest that the functional unit of the liver is in the form of an acinus. The simple liver acinus is a group of hepatocytes with its axis on the portal triad rather than around the central vein. There are three relatively discrete circulatory zones within each acinus based on the distance of cells from the supply of fresh blood from the hepatic artery. The cells receiving fresh blood (zone 1) tend to be close to the portal triad and those with the poorest supply (zone 3) tend to be near the central vein. Thus, classical anatomical descriptions of periportal centrilobular and midzonal locations, although functionally incorrect, are not incompatible with the functional liver acinus and they still form the basis of most descriptions of hepatotoxicity. The lobular, rather than the acinar concept of liver structure will be used to illustrate the principles of hepatotoxicity for the pragmatic reason that it is easier to illustrate.

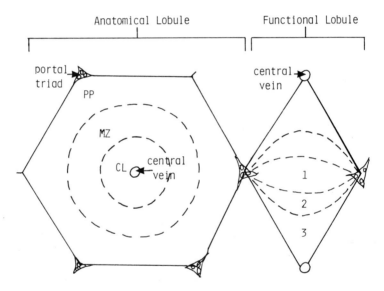

Figure 3.18. Anatomical and functional concepts of liver lobules. CL = Centrilobular; MZ = Midzonal; PP = Periportal. 1,2,3 are perfusion zones of the functional lobule.

The second major component in morphological classification of hepatic injury is the type of effect observed. This, as in all tissues, depends on the nature of the chemical and on the extent and duration of exposure, and can be any combination of degeneration, proliferation and inflammation. The type of effect also varies between species and to illustrate the principles of hepatotoxicity, the following account, based on specific types of response, is necessarily rather simplistic. The emphasis is on the more acute parenchymal lesions because these have been the focus of most studies of hepatotoxicity.

Liver hypertrophy

One of the major functions of the liver is to concentrate, biotransform and elim- inate xenobiotics. Like any other organ it will increase its capability to perform a function if demands are excessive as they often are when large amounts of chemicals are administered to animals in toxicity studies. The most frequent adap- tive response is to chemicals that are metabolised before elimination. Phenobar- bital is the classic prototype, but hundreds of chemicals fall into this category and they have the common property of a non-polar region in the molecule which permits lipid solubility at physiological pH. Elimination of such molecules is more efficient if they are converted to more polar substances and the liver will increase its functional capability if demands for such conversion exceed its normal capacity.

This functional adaptation occurs at three levels, induction or enhancement of metabolising enzymes, proliferation of organelles, notably smooth endoplasmic reticulum (SER), and the proliferation of whole cells. Enzyme induction usually involves one or more classes of cytochrome P-450 species, but other enzymes such as epoxide hydrase or glucuronyltransferases associated with the microsomal mono-oxygenases may also be induced. These xenobiotic metabolising enzymes are associated with SER primarily in the centrilobular hepatocytes. SER prolifera- tion therefore occurs mainly in the centre of the lobule. This is most clearly observed by electron microscopy as an accumulation of smooth membranous pro- files in the hepatocyte cytoplasm. By light microscopy this appears as centrilobular hypertrophy. The centrilobular hepatocytes are enlarged, the normal basophilic clumps of rough endoplasmic reticulum (RER) are dispersed and the cytoplasm may assume a very fine pale vesicular or granular eosinophilic appearance, sometimes described as 'ground-glass cytoplasm'. Glycogen storage vacuoles are reduced or absent. The nucleus is frequently enlarged and has a prominent nucleolus (Figure 3.19). The increase in cell size leads to enlargement of the whole lobule. With low doses of chemicals such as phenobarbitone, hepatocellular hyper- trophy may be the only response observed histologically. Other chemicals such as butylated hydroxytoluene may also induce numerous cell divisions and mitotic figures may be frequent in the lobule as evidence of this hyperplastic response. The increase in cell size and cell numbers often leads to an obvious increase in liver weight, particularly in rodents.

The relative contribution of cellular hypertrophy and hyperplasia to the increased liver weight is usually undetermined for most chemicals, but can be assessed by measuring DNA content. Hyperplasia will increase the total amount of DNA in the whole organ and hypertrophy will reduce the number of nuclei per unit volume and hence the amount of DNA per unit weight of liver. In rodents, liver weight is almost as sensitive an indicator of adaptation as ultrastructural evaluation or measurement of cytochrome P-450.

Increased liver weight is a very common effect in toxicity studies. It is usually considered a physiological adaptation if it is dose related, reaches a steady state with continued dosing, is reversible after cessation of treatment and is not

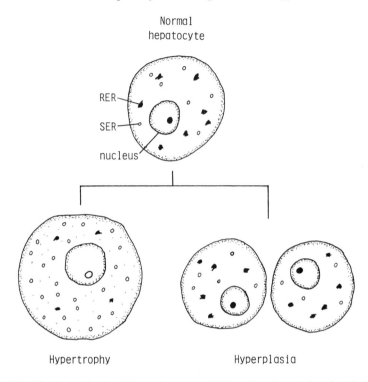

Figure 3.19. Histological basis of liver enlargement. RER = Rough endoplasmic reticulum; SER = Smooth endoplasmic reticulum.

associated with marked changes in serum enzyme levels or other measures of hepatocyte integrity. However, it is not necessarily harmless. In some cases enzyme induction may be a form of compensatory repair at the molecular level. For example, in rats the metabolism of compounds such as safrole may produce highly reactive intermediates which form ligand complexes with cytochrome P-450 and inhibit enzyme activity. This loss of P-450 activity stimulates compensatory enzyme synthesis and the subsequent metabolism of safrole leads to further ligand complex formation. The metabolism of safrole and similar precursors of reactive intermediates is thus a cycle of enzyme inhibition and induction rather than simple induction. It is important to identify this type of compensatory induction because with continued chemical administration enzyme induction gradually disappears and regressive changes appear such as distended hypoactive SER, myelin figures, lipofuscin pigment and single-cell necrosis. An analogous situation may occur in man with drugs such a phenacetin and aminophenazone. Under certain conditions of chronic analgesic administration, focal cytoplasmic degradation of SER eventually leads to pigment deposition. This pigmentation in hypertrophic hepatocytes should be taken as a signal of drug-induced injury to subcellular organelles.

Another potentially harmful effect of enzyme induction is that on the rate and route of metabolism of other chemicals. Xenobiotic enzyme inducers may enhance rates of degradation of endogenous hormones such as sex hormones and thyroid hormones. Normally, this is compensated by increased production, but where compensatory mechanisms are insufficient, hormonal imbalance may develop. The metabolism of exogenous chemicals such as carcinogens may also be enhanced. The enhancement may favour toxification or detoxification depending on a number of factors. Finally, enzyme induction may consume considerable amounts of oxygen and co-factors required for normal intermediary metabolism. This is of little consequence in healthy livers, but in disease states may exaggerate a pre-existing condition. In summary, the enzyme induction and liver enlargement that is so frequently encountered in toxicity studies is not necessarily a harmless adaptation response. Without additional information, it is not necessarily predictive of the potential effects of long-term chronic administration of xenobiotics.

Steatosis

This condition, also known as fatty change, is the accumulation of fat in the liver. A fatty liver is defined biochemically by a lipid content greater than 5% by weight and histochemically by the presence of excess fat stainable by fat-soluble dyes such as Oil red O or Sudan black. Histologically, steatosis may appear in two main forms , microvesicular and macrovesicular (Figure 3.20). In microvesicular steatosis, produced by agents such as tetracycline, the fat doplets are small, dispersed through the cytoplasm and the nucleus remains near the centre of the cell. Other chemicals such as ethanol and ethionine produce macrovesicular steatosis in which a few large fat droplets displace the nucleus towards the periphery of the cell. In terms of zonal distribution, steatosis is usually centrilobular, or, less commonly, periportal. The latter tends to occur after treatment with chemicals primarily affecting protein synthesis, whereas centrilobular steatosis is usually seen with most other toxins.

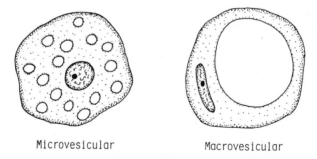

Microvesicular   Macrovesicular

Figure 3.20. Basic types of hepatocellular steatosis.

Fat is a general term for an ester or an amide of fatty acids. This is a broad definition and unless otherwise specified, steatosis or fatty liver produced by toxins refers to triglyceride accumulation which is the most frequently encountered material. Much of the current research into causal mechanisms of hepatic steatosis centres around disruption of the normal operation of the triglyceride cycle. This consists of four basic components: release, uptake, transformation and export of triglyceride-related materials (Figure 3.21). In summary, free fatty acids (FFA) are constantly released from adipose tissue triglyceride depots and transported as albumin-bound FFA to the liver, where they are either oxidised or resynthesised to triglycerides (TG). These triglycerides, together with other lipid materials are then combined with a carrier apoprotein (AP) and secreted into the blood as very low density lipoproteins (VLDLP) or as other lipoprotein species.

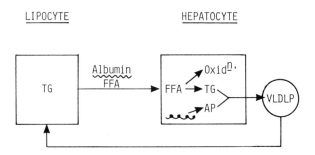

Figure 3.21. Main components of triglyceride cycle.

Chemicals may affect one or more components of the triglyceride cycle and if the imbalance is extensive, triglycerides will accumulate in the hepatocyte. In terms of the concept of extracellular and intracellular mechanisms of toxicity, triglycerides may accumulate because of extrahepatic effects causing increased supply of FFA to the liver (indirect toxicity) or because of intrahepatic disruption of triglyceride synthesis and release (direct toxicity).

Increased supply is usually due to the release of FFA from triglyceride depots in lipocytes. This is mediated by a local lipase which in turn is modulated by intracellular levels of cyclic AMP. Lipocyte cyclic AMP activity and FFA release may be enhanced by stimulation of adenylcyclase or inhibition of cyclic AMP-phosphodiesterase. Hormones of the pituitary–adrenal axis such as ACTH, corticosteroids, adrenalin and noradrenalin are the main stimulators of adenylcyclase. These stress-related hormones probably play a major role in the fatty livers associated with non-specific chemical stress or with the markedly reduced food intake sometimes seen in intoxicated animals and in animals chronically ill for other reasons such as pituitary tumours. Increased FFA release through inhibition of cyclic AMP phosphodiesterase is classically associated with methylxanthines such as caffeine and theophylline. Because the hormones and chemicals are affecting extrahepatic sites, this steatosis due to extrahepatic causes has little initial effect on liver function. However, chronic accumulation of large fat droplets may ultimately compromise liver function by decreasing the functional cytoplasmic mass of each individual hepatocyte and hence of the total liver.

Intrahepatic disruption of tryglyceride metabolism has been described with many chemicals and extensively studied with agents such as carbon tetrachloride and ethionine. The potential mechanisms for disruption are diverse, but for most chemicals are still speculative. In principle, there may be effects on critical pathways of FFA-TG metabolism, on apoprotein synthesis, or on lipoprotein synthesis and excretion. These effects may be primary chemical interaction with the critical pathways or non-specific effects secondary to chemical disruption of other hepatocellular components or metabolic routes. These primary and secondary intracellular mechanisms of hepatotoxicity are sometimes referred to as direct and indirect mechanisms of cytotoxicity. This terminology should not be confused with the use in this book of direct and indirect for intracellular and extracellular mechanisms of toxicity.

Disruption of intrahepatic FFA-TG metabolism has been associated with many chemicals, notably alcohol. Ethanol is metabolised to acetaldehyde by alcohol dehydrogenase with NAD^+ as the electron acceptor. Extensive ethanol oxidation may increase intrahepatic $NADH/NAD^+$ ratio to such an extent that the shift in redox potential affects other pathways of intermediary metabolism. Prime candidates are decreased fatty acid oxidation and the stimulation of synthesis and esterification of fatty acids, the combined effects of which would increase intracellular TG levels. However, ethanol may also affect other aspects of the triglyceride cycle such as protein synthesis and lipoprotein assembly via the potential toxic effects of excess acetaldehyde production. The precise mechanism of ethanol-induced fatty liver, if in fact there is a single mechanism, therefore remains uncertain.

With many other chemicals, investigation of the mechanism of steatosis has centred around a decrease in output of lipoproteins resulting in intracellular triglyceride accumulation. There are various potential mechanisms by which lipoprotein output may be blocked. Apoprotein production may be blocked by inhibitors of protein synthesis. For example, dimethylnitrosamine is postulated to act by alkylation of DNA and RNA. Alpha-amanitin inhibits protein synthesis due to specific blockage of RNA. The steatogenic effect of D-galactosamine is associated with sequestration of the RNA nucleotide precursor uridine 5-triphosphate (UTP). Another powerful steatogen, ethionine in the form of adenosyl-S-ethionine, inhibits amino acid incorporation into microsomal proteins by trapping the ATP required to activate the amino acids. In contrast to these relatively specific metabolic inhibitors of protein synthesis, chemicals such as CCl_4 may act non-specifically by destroying microsomal membranes through lipid peroxidation.

The drawback to the protein inhibition hypothesis is that there is often a large discrepancy between the inhibitory activity of a chemical and its potency as a steatogen and other means of blocking lipoprotein secretion have been sought. Inhibition of VLDLP assembly has been suggested for fatty liver development in orotic acid and yellow phosphorus poisoning. Depression of the hepatic secretory mechanism by effects on microtubules or membranes has been proposed for the hepatotoxicologists' favourite chemical CCl_4. Overall, the available data from compounds such as CCl_4 and ethionine suggest that multiple complex events occur both in the cell and also in extrahepatic sites and the search for specific steatogenic molecular mechanisms may be fruitless in many cases.

Necrosis (Figure 3.22)
Liver cell death may be caused by a number of drugs and chemicals. As a rule, the necrosis is of a coagulative type characterised by shrunken hypereosinophilic hepatocytes with degenerating nuclei. The extent and location of necrosis ranges from single cell to the necrosis of whole lobes (panlobular, lobar, massive). With many hepatotoxins necrosis is zonal, and often centrilobular. With other chemicals, particularly those causing unpredictable, non-dose dependent liver injury in man, the necrosis is often multifocal and scattered throughout the liver. Chemicals producing both focal and zonal necrosis may produce severe liver dysfunction if effects are widespread.

The sequel to acute hepatocellular injury is inflammation and repair. Dead cells are removed by macrophages and regenerative proliferation of remaining viable hepatocytes restores the integrity of the lobule. If the basement membranes and other supporting structures are intact, the lobule will rapidly be restored to normal. In rodents, this repair is so rapid that even extensive damage caused by potent toxins such as CCl_4 may be reversed within 14 days after a single dose. This has major implications in the conduct of acute toxicity studies. Current practice is to necropsy rodents 14 days after a single dose. Simple parenchymal cell degenerations in the liver and in many other organs will repair by regeneration during this period and be undetectable at necropsy and histologically. If the injury includes the mesenchymal supporting stroma, this will incite fibrotic repair as in any other tissue and the distortion and scarring will be detectable for some time after injury.

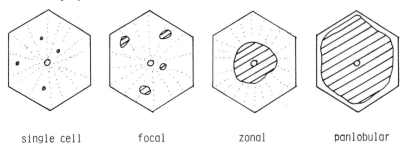

single cell   focal   zonal   panlobular

Figure 3.22. Range of acute hepatocellular necrosis.

The more detailed molecular and subcellular events associated with hepatocellular death have been extensively studied. Unfortunately, distinction between the primary molecular mechanisms associated with cell death and secondary non-specific events is still far from clear in many cases. However, the intensive study of hepatocellular death has undoubtedly yielded a considerable body of knowledge on which to base mechanistic hypotheses of toxicity for chemicals such as paracetamol and halothane.

Paracetamol produces centrilobular necrosis in a predictable dose-dependent manner due to the direct cytotoxicity of a minor metabolite thought to be *N*-acetyl-*p*-benzoquinone imine. After low doses, this *N*-hydroxylation derivative is detoxified by conjugation or by reaction with glutathione. However, after overdoses, the available glutathione is depleted and the reactive metabolite binds covalently to cellular macromolecules leading to cell death.

In man, multiple exposures to halothane may produce a mild reversible centrilobular necrosis, and more rarely a massive necrosis. In contrast to paracetamol it is not predictable and can only be reproduced with difficulty in animal models. Halothane may be metabolised by both oxidative and reductive pathways. It is suggested that reductive metabolism produces a reactive metabolite which causes the mild centrilobular necrosis by either covalent binding to critical macromolecules or via lipid peroxidation. In the rare cases of massive necrosis, it is suggested that the reactive intermediate is formed by the oxidative metabolic pathway and combines with cell membrane macromolecules to incite immune injury. Halothane is a good example of the complexity that may be found when investigating mechanisms of chemical injury. Both direct and indirect mechanisms have been implicated and these occur in an unpredictable manner.

Cholestasis

Cholestasis is the impairment of bile flow. The term was originally coined by histopathologists to indicate stagnation of bilirubin, one of the constituents of bile, in the biliary passages and hepatocytes. Bilirubin deposits are visible microscopically as green-brown pigment granules or plugs. Mechanistically, there may be several ways in which bile flow may be impaired such as physical obstruction of the bile duct or a secretory abnormality in the liver cell. The histopathologist, however, will generally see one of two basic patterns of change. These are canalicular (bland) cholestasis and cholangiolitic cholestasis (Figure 3.23). Canalicular cholestasis is classically associated with steroid contraceptives or C-17-alkylated anabolic steroids. These compounds inhibit bile secretory function selectively with little or no evidence of cytotoxicity. The histological picture is centrilobular bile plugs in an otherwise normal liver. In cholangiolitic cholestasis, produced by chemicals such as chlorpromazine, the centrilobular bile plugs are accompanied by other histological changes such as swollen or hydropic hepatocytes and periportal inflammatory reactions (cholangiolitis). In some cases, the hepatocellular degeneration is a significant feature of the overall lesion and bile stasis associated with significant degeneration and inflammation is often referred to as mixed cytotoxic/cholestatic injury.

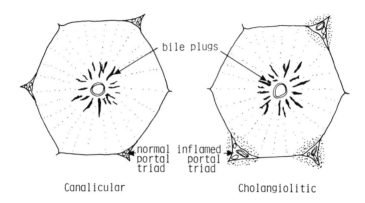

Figure 3.23. Basic types of cholestasis.

The molecular mechanisms of cholestatic injury are largely unknown and most hypotheses are based on current views of the uptake, transformation and excretion of the various components of bile. This situation is analogous to the disruption of the triglyceride cycle by chemicals causing steatosis. The major determinants of biliary secretion are bile acids. These are actively transported from blood into the hepatocyte across the sinusoidal pole of the cell by a coupling mechanism using sodium and Na^+, K^+-ATPase. Once within the hepatocyte the bile acids are transported from the sinusoidal to the canalicular pole by an undetermined mechanism. The mechanism of secretion into the canalicular lumen is also unknown. It may be by passive diffusion down an electrochemical gradient or involve carrier molecules. Other important components of the biliary micelle such as cholesterol and phospholipid are also excreted by unknown mechanisms. The accumulation of bile acids and other negatively charged solutes in the canalicular lumen results in passive movement of water and counter-ions into the lumen. This whole process is referred to as bile-acid-dependent flow. A second component of bile flow is not dependent on bile acid secretion as an osmotic force. This bile-acid-independent flow also uses Na^+, K^+-ATPase and probably accounts for about half of the usual bile flow.

Other important factors in biliary secretion are lobular gradients, the hepatocyte cytoskeletal network and resorptive processes in the ductules and ducts. Under normal basal conditions periportal (acinar zone 1) hepatocytes remove the majority of bile acid anions from the sinusoidal blood. Therefore centrilobular cells secrete bile relatively deficient in bile acids and bile-acid-independent secretion is dominant. This lobular gradient could be an important factor contributing to the commonly encountered centrilobular distribution of bile stasis as bile acids are important for solubilising lipids and other insoluble solutes. The cytoskeleton, particularly actin-containing microfilaments and the thicker microtubules, is

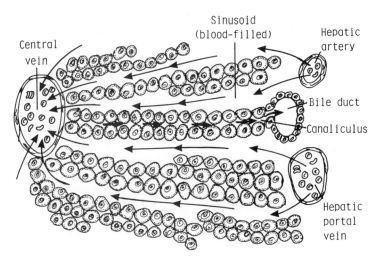

Figure 3.24. Schematic representation of sinusoidal blood and canalicular bile flow.

important to the polarity and structural integrity of the canalicular membrane. Cytoskeleton contraction may play a significant role in propelling bile along the canaliculus towards the bile ductule (Figure 3.24). Chemicals that affect the cytoskeleton may be expected to have an effect on bile flow. Finally, bile ducts and ductules are not passive structures and further water or ionic changes, notably resorption, may concentrate luminal bile fluid components to toxic levels or cause precipitation. This is analogous to the concentrating effect along the distal nephron of the kidney.

It should be apparent from the above discussion that present knowledge of normal bile secretion is sketchy and that hypotheses of chemically induced impairment by steroids, chlorpromazine and other substances are necessarily speculative. Steroid-induced canalicular cholestasis is largely predictable, dose dependent and reproducible in experimental animals. In rats, the bile-acid-independent fraction of secretion is inhibited. There is also inhibition of Na^+, K^+-ATPase, a profound alteration of membrane lipid composition, a marked increase in biliary permeability to sucrose and morphological changes in the canalicular membrane such as altered microvilli and pericanalicular microfilaments. Which, if any, of these is critical to impairment of bile flow is unknown.

There are two aspects to the toxicity of phenothiazines such as chlorpromazine. First, there is a predictable dose-dependent minor liver abnormality in man, and several dose-dependent effects can be demonstrated in experimental models. Secondly, chlorpromazine produces a more severe unpredictable form of injury in a few patients. Chlorpromazine undergoes an enterohepatic circulation and is highly concentrated in bile. In addition, it is an amphipathic cationic tertiary amine detergent that may interdigitate with lipid bilayers and disrupt membrane function and pericanalicular cytoskeletal elements. The compound is also actively metabolised and the dihydroxy derivative is a potent inhibitor of membrane Na^+, K^+-ATPase. There is also the possibility that free radicals may be generated and damage membrane lipids. These and other biochemical studies indicate that chlorpromazine and its metabolites have marked effects on liver membrane function and turnover. This is supported by the ultrastructural observations of loss of canalicular microvilli, pericanalicular vacuolation and the accumulation of intralysosomal membranous whorls (myelin figures). In view of the multiplicity of these effects, it is not surprising that chlorpromazine and its metabolites have major effects on both bile acid-dependent and -independent canalicular secretion in experimental models such as isolated perfused livers. However, the relevance of these effects at the canalicular level to the ductular lesions that are associated with the 1% of patients who develop clinically significant cholangiolitic cholestasis is uncertain. This second form of chloropromazine injury in man is unpredictable, and often associated with eosinophilia and the production of anti-nuclear antibodies suggesting immune injury as a causal mechanism. These observations are yet another example of the fact that chemicals may cause tissue injury by more than one mechanism.

Hepatic porphyria

This is another condition in which pigment may be deposited in the liver. The porphyrins are nitrogen-containing, tetrapyrrolic pigments which as complexes with iron (haems) are essential components of many cytochromes and haem-containing enzymes as well as of haemoglobin. There are several steps in the synthesis of haem (Figure 3.25). The system is regulated by negative feedback of the end product on the first step of haem synthesis which is the condensation of glycine and succinyl-CoA to form δ-aminolaevulinic acid (ALA). Under certain conditions the control mechanism is disrupted and the synthesis of porphyrin precursors exceeds their conversion to haem. These precursor molecules accumulate or are excreted and this condition is known as porphyria.

Chemicals stimulate porphyrin synthesis by reducing the concentration of haem regulating the first step in haem synthesis. This reduction of regulatory haem may be achieved either by blocking one of the intermediate steps in haem synthesis, or by increasing utilisation or removal of haem. A partial block in haem synthesis is by far the most important mechanism. For example, griseofulvin inhibits the enzyme ferrochelatase and blocks the incorporation of iron into protoporphyrin to form haem. Feedback stimulation of ALA synthetase leads to excess protoporphyrin synthesis. Protoporphyrin is relatively insoluble, is excreted in the bile and precipitates at abnormally high concentrations. The precipitates are visible histologically as brown plugs in the biliary tree or as finer granules in hepatocytes and Kupffer cells. Other porphyrin precursors are water soluble and tend to be excreted in the urine. The fungicide hexachlorobenzene, for example, increases liver production and urinary excretion of uroporphyrin by inhibiting uroporphyrinogen decarboxylase.

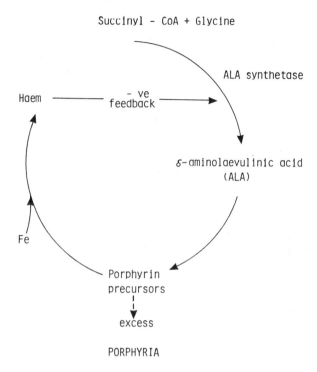

Figure 3.25. Summary of haem synthesis.

Increased porphyrin synthesis as a result of increased removal or utilisation of haem has been described with several chemicals. These chemicals, such as allyl-containing acetamides and barbiturates, usually contain unsaturated groupings and are probably converted by cytochrome P-450 to epoxides or other reactive derivatives. The active metabolites react with the haem of cytochrome P-450 and possibly with other liver haems and change its structure. This stimulates compensatory haem synthesis.

Chronic liver injury

Chronic liver injury or chronic hepatitis is a catch-all term to encompass a variety of injuries that often fail to show any uniformity with regard to their pathogenesis and histological appearance. It encompases various combinations and degrees of degeneration, proliferation, inflammation and repair. In man, there appear to be two main pathogenetic mechanisms. The first type results from the cumulation of minor cytotoxic changes caused by repeated exposure to direct cytotoxins. Isoniazid and probably alcohol are the main examples in this category. The second type has a relatively long asymptomatic latent period followed by the slow appearance of chronic liver injury. Oxyphenisatin, methyldopa and nitrofurantoin are the classic examples of this category and probably act via immune mechanisms.

Chronic liver injury produced by the tuberculostatic drug isoniazid is characterised by progressive spread of centrilobular single-cell necrosis and reparative collagen synthesis. With continued treatment, bands of fibrous tissue may form septa distorting and separating lobules, deranging the vascular supply and causing nodular hyperplasia of the surviving liver tissue. This progression to a fibrosing nodular liver is known as cirrhosis (Figure 3.26). Cirrhosis is often classified as micronodular or macronodular depending on the size of the liver nodules. Similar effects have been reported with high doses of aspirin and chronic paracetamol administration. Progression to cirrhosis is not inevitable and if exposure to drugs or chemicals is terminated, the injury subsides. This type of lesion can be reproduced in experimental animals by chronic exposure to sublethal doses of direct cytotoxins such as CCl_4. It is a predictable consequence of repeated episodes of degeneration and repair. Chronic administration of chemicals causing cholangiolitic cholestasis can also cause progressive injury. In this case destruction, regeneration and reparative fibrosis of bile ducts and adjacent hepatocytes leads to cirrhosis emanating from the periportal area. This is often termed biliary cirrhosis.

The second type of chronic liver injury seen in man is usually attributed to immune mechanisms and cannot be reproduced in laboratory animals. The pathogenesis, after an asymptomatic latent period, is similar to that of the direct cytotoxins. There is comparatively minor, but cumulative injury leading to gradual transformation of the liver architecture and ultimately cirrhosis. The process may manifest in several ways, but epithelial necrosis and cholestasis usually predominate, variably accompanied by periportal leucocyte infiltration. Injury regresses after termination of exposure, but re-exposure may provoke strong reactions.

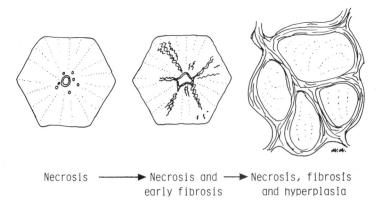

Necrosis ⟶ Necrosis and ⟶ Necrosis, fibrosis
early fibrosis   and hyperplasia

Figure 3.26. Development of cirrhosis following chronic liver injury.

Kidney

The kidney is a frequent target for the toxic action of chemicals. The main reasons for its susceptibility are related to the large fluid transfers associated with elimination of waste products and xenobiotics and with body water, electrolyte and acid–base homeostasis. To achieve these solute and water transfers, the kidney contains thousands of nephrons. Each nephron consists of a complex epithelium in intimate association with a complex blood supply (Figure 3.27).

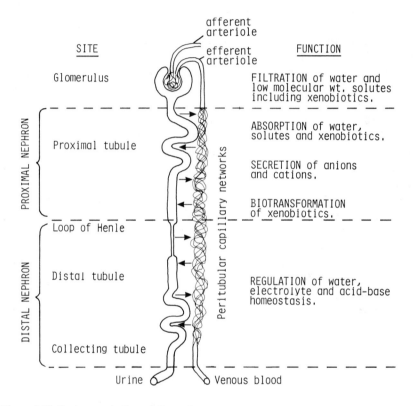

Figure 3.27. Basic organisation of the nephron.

The fluid exchanges associated with renal function mean that the kidney requires a large blood supply. The two kidneys together receive about 25% of the cardiac output and hence are exposed to larger quantities of potential toxins than most other organs. In addition, the kidney has two mechanisms which concentrate xenobiotics. Reabsorption of water from the tubule lumen may concentrate xenobiotics filtered at the glomerulus. Alternatively, active transfer of certain compounds from the plasma to the tubule lumen may lead to higher concentration in the proximal tubule cell than in the plasma. Finally, there are biotransforming enzymes capable of metabolically activating drugs and chemicals. The two main metabolising systems are cytochrome P-450 mixed function oxidases in the proximal tubule cells and prostaglandin endoperoxide synthetase in the inner medulla and renal papilla. Cytochrome P-450-mediated xenobiotic biotransformation is probably similar to that in the liver cell and may lead to the production of electrophiles or free radicals. Prostaglandin endoperoxide synthetase can co-oxygenate a variety of substances with arachidonic acid to produce reactive metabolites capable of covalently binding to cell macromolecules.

Classification of nephrotoxicity is difficult because of the complex structure of the kidney. The various epithelial and vascular elements are interdependent so that an effect in one segment frequently impacts on other areas of the nephron and the primary location of the toxicity may be difficult to define. In addition, a single chemical may affect more than one site depending on the nature and extent of exposure. Alternatively it may exert a toxic effect via more than one mechanism. In this section, the classification is based on the location and nature of the injury with a discussion of the causal mechanisms where these are known or reasonably well understood. The reader is reminded once again that classification schemes are simplifications to illustrate the principles of toxicological pathology and that the reality is often much more complicated for the reasons outlined above.

Glomerulonephropathy

The glomeruli are infrequent targets for the toxic effects of chemicals. They may be injured either directly or indirectly. A knowledge of the functional anatomy of the glomerulus is prerequisite to understanding the effects of chemicals (Figure 3.28). The glomerulus acts as a filter of plasma and consists of three main layers which produce a filtrate of virtually protein-free plasma. The glomerular capillary endothelial cells contain numerous pores (fenestrations) which allow the passage of all the non-cellular elements of the blood. The strongly anionic capillary basement membrane is continuous, but allows small molecules to permeate. Larger molecules such as albumin (68 000 MW) are retained. Cationic molecules penetrate the membrane more freely than anionic molecules of similar size. The role in the filtration process of the 25 nm slit pores between the foot processes of the epithelial cells is uncertain. The mesangial cell and associated mesangial matrix form a supporting structure for the glomerulus. The mesangium is a potential site for deposition, uptake and transport of particulate and macromolecular aggregates such as immune complexes.

Direct chemical injury to the glomerulus is uncommon (Figure 3.29). The most extensively studied example is the aminonucleoside of puromycin (6-dimethylaminopurine-3-amino-d-ribose). This causes minor lesions histologically, but ultrastructurally there is a fusion and loss of foot processes of the epithelial cells with consequent alteration of the slit pores. There are also changes in the basement membrane. The result is an increased permeability to plasma proteins which ultimately appear in the urine (proteinuria). In rats the proteinuria may

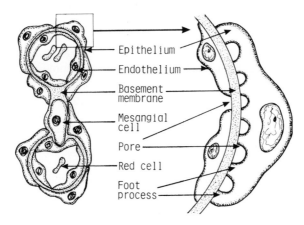

Figure 3.28. Basic organisation of the glomerular filter.

disappear and then reappear to give a clinically biphasic disease. The cause of the glomerular changes is possibly associated with a direct effect of the drugs on metabolic processes such as nucleotide synthesis in the epithelial cell.

Changes in foot processes can also be induced with charged molecules. Experimental infusion of the polycation protamine sulphate causes blunting, swelling and flattening of foot processes which is reversible by infusion of the polyanion heparin. These changes are presumably related to the highly charged nature of the basement membrane and associated structures. The highly polar cationic aminoglycoside antibiotics also effect the glomerular filter. They reduce the ultrafiltration coefficient of the glomerular filter, an effect associated with a reduction in the number and size of endothelial pores.

Immune injury may also damage the glomerulus. The precise mechanism (Types I–IV) is difficult to define, but often appears to involve immune complex deposition (Type III). d-Penicillamine, a breakdown product of penicillin has been associated with a proteinuria and nephrotic syndrome in man following its use as a chelator of metal ions for the treatment of heavy-metal poisoning. In animal experiments, there are granular deposits of immune complexes and complement along the glomerular basement membrane and in the mesangium. The glomerular alteration caused by such deposits is frequently termed glomerulonephritis, although the evidence of an inflammatory reaction is often sparse. The relationship of penicillamine to the immune complexes is uncertain since it has a low molecular weight. The appearance and effects of immune complex deposition is highly variable. It may present as focal or diffuse inflammatory lesions, both transient or progressive and also as thickening of the glomerular loops depending on the concentration and duration of complexes in the blood, their size and rate of deposition.

Continued administration of low doses of mercury preparations such as diuretics or in ointments occasionally produces an immune-mediated glomerulonephropathy and proteinuria. This can also be produced experimentally in certain strains of rat. In these experimental models, the disease is biphasic with initial deposits of antibasement membrane antibodies followed by deposition of immune complexes. The role played by mercury as an antigen is unknown. It may directly act as a hapten or indirectly alter endogenous molecules to induce an autoimmune disease.

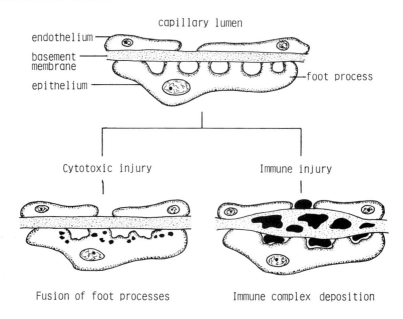

Figure 3.29. Forms of glomerulonephropathy leading to altered permeability and proteinuria.

Proximal tubular nephropathy

The proximal tubule is the most common site of nephrotoxicity. It usually consists of some type of degeneration (Figure 3.30), variably accompanied by inflammatory and repair reactions depending on the nature and extent of injury. The functions of the proximal tubule include iso-osmotic reabsorption of salt and water along with other solutes such as glucose and the proteins that escape the glomerular filtering process. It also secretes material into the tubule lumen and is capable of biotransforming many xenobiotics. All these tubular processes are dependent on an intimate relationship with the peritubular vasculature and thus there are several potential targets for both direct and indirect chemical injury.

Hydropic change

Increased fluid in the proximal tubular cell cytoplasm may occur in the early phases of degenerations leading to necrosis. It may also be seen as a distinct endpoint with various chemicals. A vacuolation of the convoluted tubule termed 'osmotic

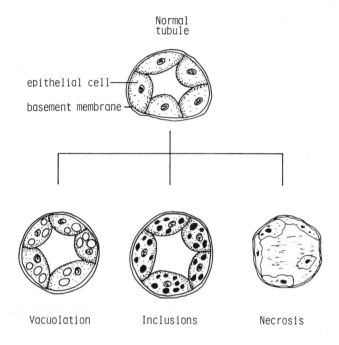

Figure 3.30. Degenerations of the proximal tubular epithelium.

nephrosis', occurs after injections of hypertonic glucose, saccharose, inulin or gelatin. These vacuoles are probably pinocytotic vacuoles containing substrate and water absorbed from the tubule lumen and represent a physiological effect rather than a true toxic degeneration. In man, vacuolation has also been associated with long-standing potassium depletion of various causes. In some cases this represents secondary toxicity rather than a primary effect, loss of potassium in enteric conditions or following chronic laxative abuse being prime examples.

Inclusions

These may occur in either nucleus or cytoplasm. Metals such as lead, cadmium and mercury will alter nuclear function in proximal tubule cells. Continued lead accumulation will cause the formation of eosinophilic intranuclear inclusion bodies. Cytoplasmic inclusions are a more frequently encountered effect of chemicals. Chronic oestrogen administration for example, produces large brown pigment granules in the proximal tubular epithelium of the rat. Inclusions due to lysosomal storage of polar lipids can be induced in experimental animals by chronic administration of various amphiphilic cationic drugs such as the anorexigenic agent chlorphentermine. Ultrastructurally, these inclusions consist of multilamellar aggregates of lipid membranes. Finally, eosinophilic globules due to lysosomal accumulation of protein (hyaline droplets) are sometimes seen. The renal proximal tubule absorbs by endocytosis the low molecular weight proteins filtered in the glomerulus. These are catabolised by lysosomal proteolytic enzymes and re-utilised. Chemicals accumulating in lysosomes or interfering with lysosomal enzymes may inhibit catabolism and lead to the intralysosomal accumulation of proteins. The male rat appears particularly prone to hyaline droplet formation. If accumulation continues, the cell may die and the appearance resembles acute tubular necrosis.

Necrosis

Necrosis of proximal tubular epithelium is the most frequently encountered form of nephrotoxicity, at least in experimental animals receiving high doses of new chemical entities. Cell injury may occur via a variety of mechanisms and may range from superficial injury to injury extending beyond the basement membrane to affect the supporting stroma (interstitium). The pathology follows the same basic pattern described in Chapter 2. Cells shrink and die and are shed into the tubule lumen. If injury extends beyond the basement membrane it will incite an inflammatory reaction. Repair will occur via epithelial regeneration or, with more extensive tubular damage, by a combination of regeneration and fibrosis. Aminoglycoside antibiotics, heavy metals, halogenated hydrocarbons and a few other examples are briefly described to illustrate the various mechanisms in proximal tubular necrosis.

Aminoglycoside antibiotics such as gentamicin sometimes produce nephrotoxicity in clinical practice. Their effect on the glomerulus has already been described, but the more pronounced effect is on the proximal tubule. The effect ranges from cellular swelling through myeloid body formation to necrosis depending on the dosage and duration of exposure. The toxicity is mediated through intracellular mechanisms, but the precise pathway is unknown. Aminoglycosides exert their bacteriocidal effect by binding to specific ribosomal proteins and inhibiting protein synthesis, and it is tempting to attribute toxicity to similar mechanisms. Lysosomal accumulation of aminoglycosides may inhibit phospholipases and hydrolases and block catabolic process in the cell.

Many heavy metals produce proximal tubular necrosis. Low doses of chromium kill cells in the proximal convoluted tubule by direct action on the cell. Higher doses produce toxicity through the proximal tubule. Mercury, a much studied nephrotoxin, causes necrosis initially in the straight part of the tubule (pars recta). The precise mechanisms of injury are unknown, but probably include both direct effects on the epithelium and ischaemia due to effects on the vasculature. Cadmium nephrotoxicity is unusual in that it is associated with metallothionein, a metal-binding protein synthesised in the liver. Inorganic cadmium, unlike other heavy metals, has virtually no acute effects on the kidney except at near-lethal doses. Its effects are due to a progressive accumulation of metallothionein-bound cadmium. This eventually reaches a critical concentration, above which cell death occurs. The morphological changes are non-specific. Tubular degeneration occurs in the initial stages, progressing to an interstitial inflammatory reaction and fibrosis.

Several halogenated hydrocarbons are nephrotoxic as well as hepatotoxic, although the latter usually predominates. In these cases, necrosis is probably due to reactive metabolites generated by cytochrome P-450 in the proximal tubular epithelium. Chloroform is interesting in that male mice of certain strains are extremely sensitive.

The kidney is also susceptible to injury by extracellular or indirect mechanisms. Of these, vascular effects predominate because of the high blood flow and dual capillary bed in the kidney. In human clinical medicine acute tubular necrosis due to haemodynamic effects is quite frequent and sometimes termed 'shock kidney'. Hypovolaemic shock due to hypotension may occur with a variety of intoxications that cause severe diarrhoea or vomiting. Hypotension may also be produced by excessive administration of anti-hypertensive drugs or CNS depressants, or during narcosis. Histologically, there is a predilection for damage in the pars recta, often characterised by patchy tubular necrosis rather than the diffuse necrosis characteristic of potent direct nephrotoxins. Chemically induced intravascular haemolysis can also cause secondary acute renal failure. Haemoglobin released from the red cells is filtered at the glomerulus and aggregates in the tubular lumen (haemoglobin casts). A similar effect follows massive muscle injury, but in this case it is myoglobin casts that form in the tubules.

Immune-mediated tubular injury is not common. In main, the drugs most frequently implicated are methicillin, ampicillin, rifampicin, phenindione and sulphonamides. The precise mechanisms have not been defined. Antibodies reacting with tubular basement membrane have been found in some cases, and in others, cell-mediated immunity (Type IV) has been suggested. Morphologically, the acute lesion is a tubulointerstitial nephritis. In other words, as well as tubular injury and regeneration, there is a prominent inflammatory reaction in the interstitial stroma around the tubules. This is characterised by interstitial oedema and an inflammatory infiltrate made up predominantly of lymphocytes and plasma cells.

Distal tubular nephropathy

The tubular components of the distal nephron are the loop of Henle, the distal tubule itself and the collecting duct. They are considered together because they are concerned with the regulation of water, electrolytes and acid-base balance. The end result is a concentrated, slightly acidic urine representing about 1% of the volume filtered at the glomerulus. The most frequently encountered toxic effects are crystalluria and renal papillary necrosis.

Crystalluria

Chemicals or their metabolites may crystallise in the tubule lumen as they are concentrated in the distal nephron. Changes in pH may also affect the degree of ionisation and solubility of organic acids and bases and lead to crystallisation. Microcrystals may pass through the tubule with little effect. Larger ones may be irritant or mechanically injure the tubule lining and cause tubular obstruction. In these cases, the histological picture is usually widespread tubular dilatation due to obstruction, and various forms of debris in the tubule lumen such as leucocytes and dead cells, due to irritation. Sometimes the crystals themselves are visible. Most often, they dissolve during histological processing to leave cleft-like spaces surrounded by tubular epithelial cells or multinucleate phagocytic cells. The tubular lesions are frequently accompanied by an interstitial inflammatory reaction (Figure 3.31). Crystalluria is classically associated with sulphonamides and with ethylene glycol. Crystallisation of sulphonamides is due to a combination of concentration and a change in solubility caused by pH changes. In the case of ethylene glycol, the crystals are calcium oxalate resulting from metabolism of the parent glycol.

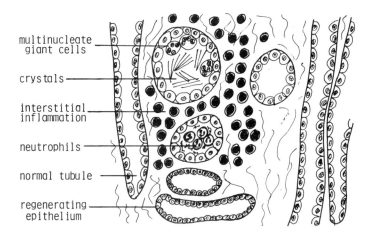

Figure 3.31. Tubulointerstitial reaction to irritant crystals.

Renal papillary necrosis (RPN)

This is a major cause of chronic renal failure in man accounting for well over 10% of cases in many surveys of renal disease. It is associated with chronic analgesic abuse and mixtures of analgesics such as aspirin and phenacetin are more toxic than the individual drugs. RPN can also be produced experimentally by both acute and long-term administration of analgesic and non-steroid anti-inflammatory compounds.

There are probably three or more stages in the development of the lesion: focal necrobiosis, intermediate or partial papillary necrosis and advanced or total papillary necrosis (Figure 3.32). The early focal necrobiosis is an interstitial lesion at the tip of the papilla. There are patchy necroses of the interstitial cells, capillaries and loops of Henle accompanied by changes in the interstitial matrix supporting these structures. The collecting ducts are normal. In the intermediate stage the necrosis extends to affect more of the papilla, but the collecting ducts are little affected. Finally, in advanced cases the total papilla is necrotic and sharply demarcated from the outer medulla, or detached from it. There are secondary changes in the cortex such as tubular atrophy, degeneration or dilatation accompanied by interstitial fibrosis and a variable mononuclear leucocyte infiltration. This is termed chronic interstitial nephritis.

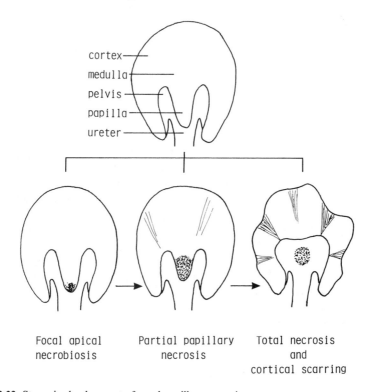

Figure 3.32. Stages in development of renal papillary necrosis.

The pathogenesis of RPN is controversial. There is little disagreement that the earliest changes occur at the tip of the papilla and affect the renal concentrating mechanisms as a primary factor. However, opinion is divided concerning the structures initially affected. The primary cause may be via vascular injury either by direct cytotoxicity to vascular endothelium or vasoconstriction due to inhibition of the synthesis of the renal vasodilator prostaglandin E. Cytotoxic effects on the loop of Henle or interstitial cells may also play a role in the genesis of the lesion. Overall, RPN probably results from the combined effects of direct cellular toxicity and medullary ischaemia in areas where the chemical or a metabolite is concentrated.

Nervous system

The nervous system is of fundamental importance in maintaining body homeostasis. It receives signals both from the external and from the internal environment and modifies body function accordingly. It is a highly complex and specialised system, one or more parts of which may be susceptible to chemical injury. The ways in which the functional specialisations in various parts of the system make it vulnerable to injury are illustrated with examples from the central and peripheral nervous system and from two of the special sense organs: eye and ear.

Central and peripheral nervous system (CNS/PNS)

Both pharmacokinetic and pharmacodynamic elements influence the selective sensitivity of the nervous system to toxic insult. The main pharmacokinetic element is the so-called blood–brain barrier which prevents the entry of certain chemicals into the nervous system. Neurovascular endothelium, unlike that in other vessels, is not fundamentally porous. The cells are linked by tight junctions which effectively seal off intercellular transport of macromolecules. In addition, transcellular transport via pinocytosis is also less active than in other tissues. A further potential barrier is the complex network of astrocytic foot processes which surround the capillaries of the CNS. An equivalent barrier is present in much of the PNS. The neurovascular endothelium thus presents as a continuous highly lipophilic membrane which excludes most polar molecules from the neural tissue. However, non-polar lipid-soluble molecules such as solvents and anaesthetics will penetrate the nervous system with ease. A further pharmacokinetic difference between neural tissue and other tissues is the general paucity of toxicant metabolising systems. This may be disadvantageous or advantageous depending on whether the parent compound or metabolite is the primary toxic molecule.

The pharmacodynamic elements affecting selective sensitivity are complex because the nervous system consists of many cell types with different functions and hence different biochemical targets for attack by toxicants. However, the neurone is generally considered to be the most sensitive cell because of the glucose-dependent high metabolic activity associated with active ion transport. Also, the neurone has very long processes which have to be supported by synthetic processes in the cell body and by sophisticated transport systems.

Overall, the nervous system is selectively protected from polar chemicals by the blood – neural barrier and at the same time vulnerable to the effects of chemicals that can cross this barrier. As many chemicals, particularly drugs, are designed to cross lipid barriers to improve absorption from the gastrointestinal tract, and because neurologically active compounds are of intense therapeutic interest, it is not surprising that neurological responses should be fairly common in regulatory toxicity studies. The types of clinical response that may be seen include hyperactivity, tremors, convulsions, sedation and paralysis. These and many other behavioural responses can be divided into two main groups. The type most frequently encountered is the acute, transient, reversible response that is not accompanied by any obvious light microscopic changes in the nervous system. This type of response is common in short-term, high-dose studies and is usually classified as a pharmacological effect. The second type of response is the permanent or slowly reversible behavioural change that is often accompanied by morphological change in the nervous system. Such responses are classified as toxic effects, and it is this category that is reviewed in this section.

The main type of toxic response observed histologically is degeneration. However, the structure and composition of the nervous system is complex and an equally complex language is required to describe the precise location and nature of any lesion. Fortunately, much of this can be reduced to a reasonably basic level to illustrate the principles of neurotoxicity. These basic principles are derived from an understanding of the basic organisational anatomy of the nervous system. It consists essentially of three components: nerve cells, supporting cells and vascular tissue (Figure 3.33). The neurone consists of cell body (soma), cell processes (axon, dendrites) and the synaptic zones used in neurotransmission. The two main supporting cells are the myelin-producing cells and astrocytes. Oligodendrocytes are the myelin-producing cells of the CNS and Schwann cells myelinate the axons of the PNS. Astrocytes are a major supporting cell in the CNS and are characterised by numerous processes interspersed between the other neural elements and around blood vessels. In the CNS, the oligodendrocytes, astrocytes and microglia (phagocytes) are collectively known as glial cells. The neurovascular component has already been discussed in relation to the blood–brain barrier but it is an important target site of certain neurotoxins.

Any one or a combination of these component sites can be the target for toxic

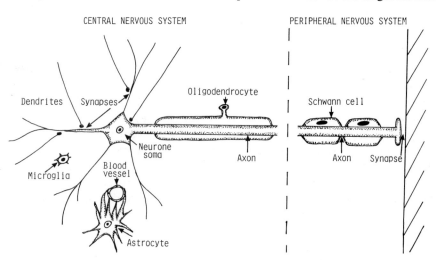

Figure 3.33. Basic organisation of CNS and PNS illustrated by a motor neurone.

chemicals. The primary classification of pathological responses in the nervous system is derived by combining the site of toxicity with the suffix -opathy (Table 3.1). Each primary lesion can be subclassified on the basis of qualifying terms specifying the location of the lesion more precisely. For example, an axon lesion near the cell body may be referred to as a proximal axonopathy and one near the nerve ending as a distal axonopathy. The location of the axon in the CNS or PNS can also be included as a qualifying term using the terms central and peripheral respectively. Thus, a central distal axonopathy refers to lesions of axon endings in the CNS. Similarly, synaptopathy may be defined as a pre- or post-synaptic lesion. Finally, qualifying terms such as sensory and motor may be used to specify the functional status of the affected cell or cell process. This build-up of qualifying terms can lead to complex diagnoses such as 'sensory-motor central-peripheral distal axonopathy', meaning lesions of the distal axons of both sensory and motor neurones in the central and peripheral nervous systems.

Table 3.1. Classification of neuropathological lesion according to cell type and location.

Neurone body	Neuronopathy	Sensory, motor
Axon	Axonopathy	Proximal, distal, central, peripheral
Synapse	Synaptopathy	Pre-, post-
Oligodendrocyte ⎫ Schwann cell ⎭	Myelinopathy	
Astrocyte	Astrocytic gliopathy	
Vasculature	Neurovasculopathy	

The terminology used so far has merely specified the location of the lesion without indicating anything about the nature of the lesion. Most of the toxic lesions encountered are degenerations with variable reactions by the vascular and the glial components. Examples of the more common lesions are described below.

Neuronopathy

The neurone is highly vulnerable not only to directly cytotoxic chemicals, but also to chemicals affecting the blood and blood-flow because of the cell's critical dependence on a supply of glucose and oxygen to meet its high metabolic requirements. Acute cytotoxic or anoxic injury rapidly leads to cell death. The initial response may be cell swelling due to failure of the membrane ion transport systems, but the classical histological presentation of necrotic neurones in HE sections is as a shrunken cell with deeply eosinophilic cytoplasm lacking Nissl granules, and a pyknotic nucleus (Figure 3.34). Unfortunately, such 'dark neurones' are easily produced as artefacts and a glial response to remove the dead cell (neuronophagia) is much more convincing evidence of necrosis. Neurones cannot repair by regeneration and structural defects are repaired by proliferation of astrocytes. This is equivalent to fibrosis in other tissues and the end result is sometimes termed a 'glial scar'.

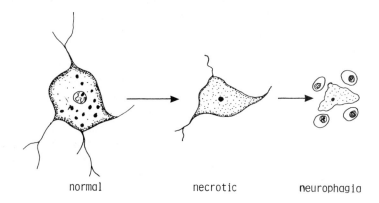

normal   necrotic   neurophagia

Figure 3.34. Acute neuronal necrosis.

Several chemicals produce neuronal necrosis. The oxygen consumption of neurones is several-fold higher than that of glial cells and the final common pathway in many cases may be anoxia. For example, neuromuscular blockers, nitrites and carbon monoxide may produce anoxic anoxia (poorly oxygenated blood). Hypotensives and vasodilators could produce ischaemic anoxia (poor blood flow), although cerebrovascular autoregulation tends to protect against such effects. Finally, cytotoxic anoxia (poor oxygen utilisation) may be produced by metabolic inhibitors such as cyanide, azide and dinitrophenol. The metabolic basis of the most studied neuronotoxin, methyl mercury, is still unknown. In the rat, this primarily affects the dorsal root ganglion cells producing focal ribosomal changes followed by nuclear lesions and ultimately death of the entire neurone. The granule cells in the cerebellum are also sensitive to the toxic effects of methyl mercury, possibly because of an effect on protein metabolism, but mercury ions also affect the blood – brain barrier and this may also play a role in the production of neuronopathy.

Not all neuronopathies are acute. Chronic sublethal injury may produce changes in subcellular organelles. Vincristine, an antimitotic alkaloid, produces a neuropathy characterised by accumulation of neurofilaments both in the neuronal perikaryon and in axons. Aluminium is also reported to produce a fibrillary change.

Axonopathy

Toxic effects on the axon, particularly in the PNS are probably the most commonly encountered neuropathy. Classical and much studied chemicals are acrylamide, carbon disulphide, n-hexane, methyl n-butyl ketone, and organophosphates. These and many other chemicals characteristically produce axonal degeneration in the distal axons of the CNS and PNS (central–peripheral distal axonopathy). The biochemical mechanism of toxicity is largely unknown, but the end result is the chemical equivalent of physical transection of the nerve resulting in what is termed Wallerian-type degeneration. If a nerve is cut physically or 'chemically', the axon distal to the cut degenerates. The associated Schwann cells contract and round up to produce myelin ovoids. The myelin-cell response is secondary to axonal degeneration, and this is known as secondary demyelination. The neuronal response to the lesion in its axon is an attempt at repair by regeneration. There is an increased synthetic activity in the cell body, characterised by cell swelling, dissolution of the basophilic clumps of Nissl substance and movement of the nucleus towards the periphery of the cell. This somal reaction is known as chromatolysis and reflects increased metabolic activity directed towards the synthesis of new axoplasm. The newly synthesised components are transported down the axon to the viable stump and accumulate as the stump sprouts to try to re-establish contact with the periphery (Figure 3.35).

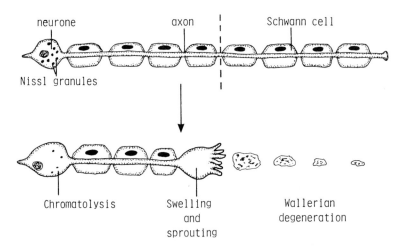

Figure 3.35. Response of a motor neurone to axon transection.

Chromatolysis, axonal swelling and Wallerian degeneration can be observed in HE-stained sections and form the basis of a neurotoxicity assay in the hen for organophosphate pesticides. The use of silver stains for axons may highlight the axonal component of the process, and myelin stains such as luxol fast blue may be used to study the secondary demyelination. At the ultrastructural level, the chemically induced distal axonopathies often fall into one of two main groups. The axonopathy caused by tri-ortho-cresyl phosphate (TOCP) is characterised by a focal or multifocal accumulation of smooth endoplasmic reticulum (SER) before the distal axon degenerates. Toxicants such as CS_2, acrylamide and hexa-carbon solvents on the other hand result in axonal swellings due to accumulation of filaments. The latter are associated with slow axonal transport mechanisms whereas SER is part of the fast axonal transport system. There is considerable interest in the biochemical mechanisms by which axonotoxins disrupt these transport processes and lead to axonal degeneration, but the precise molecular mechanisms are still unknown. Intracellular energy production may be a critical target site in many cases.

Central-peripheral distal axonopathy is the most common form of axonopathy, but other types are also known. Experimental clioquinol intoxication produces a distal axonopathy in which only the central processes of the peripheral sensory neurones degenerate. Other compounds such as β,β'-iminodipropionitrile produce a proximal axonopathy in which giant axonal swellings due to neurofilament accumulation occur in the axon regions near the cell body.

Synaptopathy

Numerous chemicals modify synaptic transmission, by interfering with synthesis, release, binding, degradation or uptake of various neurotransmitters at pre- and post-synaptic sites. In most cases there is no obvious structural alteration and such toxic responses are more amenable to the biochemical and functional assays used in neuropharmacology. Certain chemicals, however, will produce structural changes and are valuable tools in experimental neurotoxicology. Most notable are the toxic amine analogues such as 6-hydroxydopamine and 5,7-dihydroxytryptamine which cause presynaptic destruction when taken into the nerve terminal by the amine uptake receptors.

Postsynaptic destruction is less well studied, but amine analogues such as the glutamine analogue kainic acid may destroy central neurones. They act by excessive stimulation of excitatory receptors on dendrosomes and are often referred to as excitotoxins. These glutamate excitotoxins tend to act selectively in brain regions unprotected by the blood–brain barrier such as preoptic hypothalamic neurones. They cause dendrosomal swelling and ultimately cell death. Kainic acid is one of the more potent excitotoxins, but other less potent ones are potential health risks because they occur in food or are deliberately added to food. The flavouring agent monosodium glutamate is the most controversial because of its once liberal use in baby foods and its association with the 'chinese restaurant syndrome' in adults.

Myelinopathy

Myelin-producing cells are generally at less risk to toxic chemicals than neurones. However, they share one of the latter's vulnerabilities, namely a very long cell process wrapped around the axon as the myelin sheath. Myelinopathies primarily affect long axons, shorter ones often being non-myelinated. The most easily identifiable lesions in routine paraffin sections are the vacuolar or spongiform myelinopathies due to accumulation of water. These are caused by chemicals such as hexachlorophene and certain organotin compounds and the primary lesion is intramyelinic oedema. The myelin splits along the intraperiod line to produce large, fluid-filled blebs that can be seen as vacuoles by light microscopy (Figure 3.36). The milder lesions appear to be reversible, and segmental demyelination (see below) is only occasionally observed.

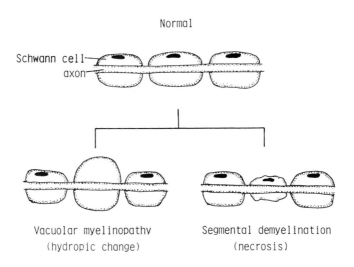

Figure 3.36. Types of myelinopathy.

A less readily detectable myelinopathy is segmental demyelination. This is seen in peripheral nerves after chronic exposure to lead or perhexiline maleate, and can also be produced by diphtheria toxin. Degeneration begins in the paranodal myelin and the node widens. At low doses, Schwann cells survive and engulf the debris, but higher doses kill the cell and myelin is lost from the whole segment covered by the Schwann cell. Adjacent cells may divide and ultimately re-myelinate the axon, but this regeneration may be imperfect producing short internodes or thin myelin sheaths in the repaired segments. Segmental demyelination is more readily observed in teased fibre preparations than in routine HE sections.

Astrocytic gliopathy

Astrocytic responses commonly accompany damage to other cellular elements, but specific astrocytic degenerations are uncommon. Methionine sulphoximine has been used as an experimental epileptic agent in mice. This chemical inhibits glutamine synthetase which is a key enzyme in handling ammonia in the brain. Astrocytes enlarge, accumulate glycogen and have large clear nuclei. These morphological changes resemble those produced by plasma ammonia levels increased either experimentally or as a result of chronic liver disease. Astroglial hypertrophy and hyperplasia is also produced by the copper chelating agent biscyclohexane oxalyldihydrazone (Cuprizone (B)) in young mice, but this also causes a concomitant oligodendroglial reaction.

Neurovasculopathy

Because of the critical dependence of neural tissue on its blood supply and the blood – brain barrier neurovasculopathy is potentially a very serious problem. This is well known in human clinical medicine in the form of 'strokes' due to haemorrhage or thrombosis in the cerebral vessels. Toxic neurovasculopathies are less well defined.

The two main pathological effects likely to be seen histologically following toxic insult to the endothelium are haemorrhage and oedema and the best known causes of such direct neurovasculopathies are the heavy metals, notably lead. Some, but not all, cases of acute lead encephalopathy in man are associated with perivascular exudates and capillary proliferation. Similar vascular lesions have been produced in suckling rodents and subhuman primates. Methyl mercury and mercuric ion are also known to injure the barrier system and oedema and haemorrhage are occasionally described in cases of intoxication. Unfortunately, such data are often overshadowed by the emphasis on the neuronal aspects of toxicity. Other metals that have been associated with cerebral haemorrhage and oedema are arsenic and bismuth, and endoneural oedema may occur in experimental tellurium toxicity in rats.

Eye

The most common toxic effects on the eye are due to surface injury. However, the eye is also at risk from chemicals administered systemically and like the brain has specialised pharmacokinetic and pharmacodynamic characteristics which make it selectively protected or selectively vulnerable to toxic chemicals. Notable among these are the blood–eye barrier, the avascular lens and retinal pigment.

Although the eye is a complex structure, it can be reduced to three basic functional components associated with phototransmission, phototransduction and neurotransmission. The majority of the globe is used in phototransmission and includes the cornea, iris, lens and vitreous humour. The lens is the main component at risk from systemically administered chemicals and the main morphological response is cataract. Phototransduction, the conversion of light energy to electrical impulses, is the province of the photoreceptor cells of the retina. These are so intimately connected with the retinal pigment epithelium and adjacent choroid that lesions often have to be considered collectively as chorioretinopathies. Retinal ganglion cells and their axons forming the optic nerve are the principal components of the neurotransmitter system and lesions can be described under the general heading of optic neuropathy.

Lens cataract

The lens is a transparent encapsulated avascular structure composed of a single cell type, the lens fibres which proliferate more or less continually throughout life. The main components are water and protein, and ionic equilibrium and protein synthesis are the main metabolic functions concerned with transparency. These in turn are totally dependent on the aqueous humour as a source of nutrients. Disturbances of proliferation or of these metabolic functions are the main mechanisms of injury. Such disturbances may occur either indirectly by altering the aqueous humour or by a direct lenticular effect. This leads to a change in refractive index to produce a translucency that is visible clinically as an opacity or 'cataract'. Cataracts are often specified by their location in the lens using qualifying terms such as subcapsular, cortical and nuclear. Chemically induced cataracts may also be classified as transient or permanent depending on the reversibility of the change.

In general, cataracts are more readily observed clinically than histologically. This is mainly due to the problem of accurately sampling focal lesions for histological section. The histological lesion may be a hydropic degeneration initiated by cell swelling and followed by rupture of the lens fibre, or a coagulative necrosis with disintegration of the cytoplasmic fibrils (Figure 3.37). The acute reversible cataracts sometimes seen in short term toxicity studies in young rats and dogs are often associated with suture lines. They are possibly due to hydropic changes in lens fibres following changes in the osmolality of the aqueous humour.

A wide range of chemicals has been reported to produce permanent cataracts

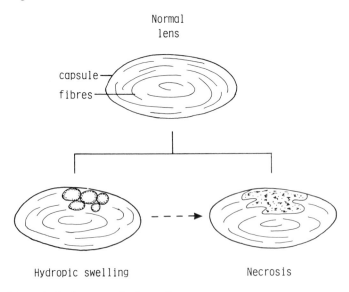

Figure 3.37. Schematic development of subcapsular cataracts.

in humans or laboratory animals, but there is often a wide variation in species' sensitivity to particular individual chemicals. In sensitive species, the cataracts are often subcapsular and frequently associated with lens sutures. In most cases, the mechanism of cataractogenesis is ill defined, but is probably associated with effects on cell proliferation, protein metabolism, or ion transfer and cytoplasmic osmolality. The antileukaemic agent busulphan probably causes cataracts by altered cell division because cataracts tend to develop more slowly in species with the slowest lens mitotic activity. The cataracts associated with chronic steroid administration and with exposure to naphthalene vapour may be in part due to effects on fibrillar protein. Other cataractogenic chemicals are thought to act on either the energy-generating systems or associated ion pumps. For example, the effect of 2,4-dinitrophenol may be related to its ability to uncouple oxidative phosphorylation, whereas the effect of thallium may be associated with Na^+–K^+ cellular transport mechanisms.

Retinopathy

The primary photoreceptors are the retinal rods and cones. Their apical portions intermingle with the microvilli of the pigment epithelial cells which play a vital role in maintaining photoreceptor function (Figure 3.38). The nutrition of the pigment epithelium and of the photoreceptor layer is via the capillaries of the choroid. All three layers — choroid, pigment cells and photoreceptors — may be the target of systemic toxins. However, effects on one layer commonly affect the others and the end stage degenerative lesion is sometimes a chorioretinopathy.

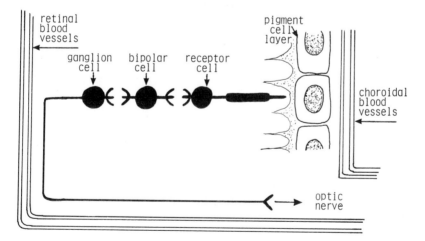

Figure 3.38. Basic structure of the retina.

Selective effects on the photoreceptor cells are uncommon, but the glycolysis inhibitor iodoacetate can produce selective damage experimentally. Many of the known retinotoxic agents appear to act primarily on the pigment epithelium or on the melanin pigment in the choroid. Such effects will not of course be detected in albino rodents. Melanin has a high binding capacity for polycyclic aromatic hydrocarbons such as chloroquine, and sufficiently high and prolonged doses may damage the pigment epithelium. Secondary responses in the photoreceptor layer result in visual impairment. Primary effects on pigment epithelium with secondary photoreceptor degeneration also occur with intravenous iodate, the antibiotic sparsomycin and certain diaminodiphenoxyalkanes. Species-specific retinopathies may occur in animals with a tapetum such as dog and rabbit. Experimental tapetal necrosis with oedema and secondary retinal degeneration, possibly due to zinc depletion, has been described following compounds such as dithizone and sodium diethylthiocarbonate. Finally, exudative retinopathies, probably reflecting primary vascular damage, can be produced by chemicals such as quinine.

Optic neuropathy

The retinal ganglion cells and their axons can be considered as a specialised form of the peripheral nervous system and are potential targets for neuronopathy, axonopathy and myelinopathy. Whilst they are at risk to chemicals causing peripheral neuropathies elsewhere in the body such as carbon disulphide, disulfiram and clioquinol, other chemicals tend to be more selective to the visual pathways than to the PNS.

Acute neuronopathy occurs in immature rodents shortly after injection of excitotoxins such as glutamate. More chronic forms of neuronopathy include accumulation of pigment in ganglion cells following chronic phenothiazine administration, and phospholipidosis with appetite-suppressant drugs such as chlorphentermine. However, these cytoplasmic accumulations are not specific to the retinal ganglion cells. Blindness associated with acute methanol poisoning is attributable, at least in part, to loss of ganglion cells. Methanol is another example of species-restricted eye lesions. Primates metabolise methanol to the proximal toxin formaldehyde via alcohol dehydrogenase whereas lower mammals favour the catalase system.

Methanol may also produce an axonopathy in primates. Oedema of the optic nerve head in monkeys seems to be associated with accumulation of material due to defective axonal transport at this site. Quinine and the antituberculous agent ethambutol are further examples of agents which preferentially affect the optic nerve, sparing the PNS, but the mechanisms are ill-defined.

Inner ear

Ototoxicity can be produced by topically applied chemicals or by chemicals administered systemically, but the term generally refers to the effects of systemically administered chemicals on the inner ear particularly the cochlea. As in the CNS, PNS and eye, the fundamental principles of ototoxicity are related to the basic organisational anatomy and physiology of the cochlea (Figure 3.39).

Much of the ear is concerned with sound conduction, but the two important components related to ototoxicity are the neural elements and the vascular elements of the inner ear. Like the eye, the neural element is composed of a transducer, the hair cell, converting physical energy to electrical impulses, and ganglion cells collecting these impulses for neurotransmission via the auditory nerve to the brain. The hair cells and associated structures form the organ of Corti. These neural elements are critically dependent on their local vascular supply, but an equally important and specialised vascular component is the stria vascularis. This structure is responsible for maintaining the fluid medium (endolymph) through which pressure waves are transmitted to the sensory hair cells. The stria vascularis is thus somewhat similar to the ciliary processes in the eye which produce aqueous humour.

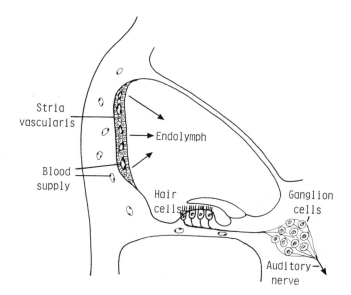

Figure 3.39. Basic organisation of the cochlear duct of the inner ear.

Ototoxic agents can theoretically act on the neural component, the vascular component or on both elements, but for many agents the precise mechanism is ill-defined. The following classification scheme using sensory neuropathy and vasculopathy is therefore subjective, but is convenient for illustrating the basic principles.

Sensory neuropathy

This is produced by agents causing primary damage to the hair cells or their associated nerve fibres. The prototype chemicals in this class are the aminoglycoside antibiotics. This is the group of drugs most apt to produce permanent deafness. The pathological response observed is degeneration, initially characterised by distortion of the cilia but eventually followed by necrosis of the whole cell. This destruction results in permanent auditory dysfunction. There are four rows of hair cells running along the cochlea, three outer and one inner. Aminoglycoside antibiotics typically damage the inner of the three rows of outer hair cells particularly those at the base of the cochlea. The resulting auditory dysfunction therefore affects sensitivity to high-frequency tones.

Similar hair cell mechanoreceptors are present in other parts of the inner ear primarily concerned with balance rather than hearing. There are several foci of such cells, collectively known as the vestibular apparatus. Aminoglycosides may also damage these cells and produce disturbances of balance and posture referred to as vestibulotoxicity. The biochemical mechanism of aminoglycoside ototoxicity is unknown. They have a strong affinity for calcium-binding membrane phospholipids and displacement of calcium or inhibition of the function of these polyphosphoinositides may disrupt membrane integrity and lead to cell death. Other theories correlate ototoxicity with aminoglycoside effects on glucose transport, carbohydrate metabolism and energy cycles.

Vasculopathy

Several chemicals produce transient or reversible auditory disturbances rather than permanent deafness. These include salicylates, other non-steroidal anti-inflammatory agents, quinine and certain loop diuretics. The mechanisms are unclear, but are possibly the results of effects on the cochlear microvasculature or the endolymph. Experimental salicylate and quinine intoxications are reported to produce endothelial swelling and partial capillary occlusion. The vascular effect of salicylates may be related to their action on prostaglandins. The locus of attack of certain arsenicals is considered to be the stria vascularis. The loop diuretics also affect the stria vascularis producing oedema, ultrastructural changes in marginal cells and changes in the ion-transporting mechanism of the stria. Such ion changes in the endolymph would affect the electrophysiological performance of the organ of Corti. Prolonged administration of loop diuretics may lead to structural damage in the stria vascularis and to cases of permanent auditory dysfunction, but a more sinister aspect is the marked synergism that occurs when loop diuretics and aminoglycosides are given together.

Cardiovascular system

The cardiovascular system like the nervous system, is one of the body's fundamental life-support systems and adverse effects on its structure and function are of critical interest in toxicology. Anatomically, it is conventially divided into the heart and blood vessels and one or both of these sites may be the target for toxic injury. The heart is particularly susceptible to some chemicals because of its high degree of specialisation.

Heart

The heart has one of the properties of the nervous system that is a potentially vulnerable target for toxins, namely cells with electrically excitable membranes. This excitable membrane, the sarcolemma, unlike that of the motor neurone is coupled to an intracellular contraction system and these two properties, excitation and contraction have high energy requirements. The heart has the highest energy demands on a weight basis of any organ in the body and this requires a continued supply of oxygen to support aerobic metabolism. Oxygen supply and utilisation is therefore a second area of vulnerability. To illustrate the principles of cardiac toxicology the heart can be reduced to an oxygen-dependent contractile cell driven by an excitable membrane that is subject to neurohumoral control (Figure 3.40).

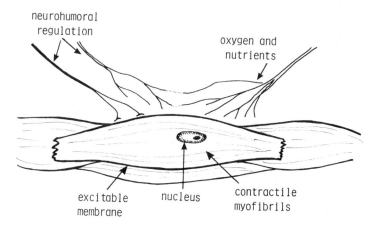

Figure 3.40. Basic organisation of cardiac muscle.

Functional effects

Cardiotoxicity is a relatively infrequent adverse reaction in humans. However, a large number of compounds of potential therapeutic value in cardiovascular or neurological disease are administered at high doses to animals in drug development studies and cardiac effects are often encountered. The vast majority of effects are acute, transient, functional responses, and reversible if the animal does not die. These functional responses include bradycardia, tachycardia and various forms of arrhythmia, and like their equivalents in the nervous system these 'cardiotoxicities' are generally considered to be exaggerated pharmacological effects.

In many of the well-studied cases of functional abnormalities the mechanism is related to effects on the ion shifts across the cell membrane (sarcolemma) that are used in the action potential. Digitalis and related cardiotonic chemicals are probably toxic by inhibiting membrane Na^+, K^+-ATPase, which maintains the normal transcellular gradients of potassium and sodium. Other chemicals disturbing ion shifts across the cell membrane are tetrodotoxin, tetraethyl ammonium and verapamil which reduce the inflow of Na^+, K^+ and Ca^{2+} respectively. Other toxins are thought to act on intracellular sites. Heavy metals such as mercurials affect mitochondrial function and may depress the energy production vital to excitation-contraction coupling. The depression of cardiac contractility by halothane may be related in part to inhibition of myosin ATPase activity. Thus, there are many potential intracellular mechanisms by which toxins may interfere with excitation–contraction coupling to produce functional abnormalities. Many cardiotoxic agents probably interfere with this process at several sites.

Cardiomyopathy

In contrast to the frequent occurrence of functional effects, relatively few cardiotoxic agents cause structural changes in the heart. When effects are noted they are usually characterised by degeneration followed by inflammation and repair. These lesions are designated as cardiomyopathies. Myocardial (cardiac) necrosis is the most frequently studied cardiomyopathy. In principle, this can result indirectly by disturbance of the blood supply to the myocyte (hypoxic injury) or by direct chemical insult to the myocyte (cytotoxic injury) or by a combination of both effects. The end result, necrosis, is essentially the same, but the location of the lesion may differ. Hypoxic injury tends to affect fairly specific sites, whereas cytotoxic injury may be more widespread (Figure 3.41).

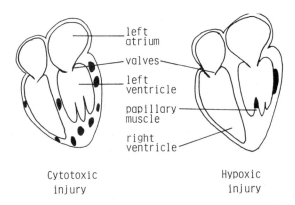

Figure 3.41. Sites of myocardial necrosis.

Bronchodilators and vasodilators are the compounds classically producing site-specific necrosis. One or a few doses of isoproterenol produce acute cardiac necrosis in rat heart with a striking tendency for the subendocardial regions at the apex of the left ventricle. The vasodilator hydralazine produces similar lesions. In beagles, the apex of the left ventricular papillary muscles is the favoured site. Continued administration does not increase the incidence or severity of the lesions and the initial acute lesions heal by fibrosis. Such acute cardiomyopathies could easily be missed in long-term studies, unless specific connective tissue stains are used to highlight the fibrosis.

The pathogenetic mechanism of this site-specific necrosis is not totally understood, but myocardial hypoxia probably plays an important role. Vasodilation may lower coronary perfusion and tachycardia increases oxygen demand. As the capillary pressure is lowest subendocardially, this area is at most risk to oxygen deprivation. The papillary muscles supporting the forces on the valves have the greatest oxygen requirement and are similarly at risk. The sites of injury are thus consistent with the hypothesis of myocardial hypoxia. As this is related to the pharmacological effects of these agents, acute cardiac necrosis produced by vasoactive drugs can be considered to be the result of an exaggerated pharmacological effect.

Myocardial hypoxia depletes intracellular high-energy phosphate stores required to maintain membrane ion shifts. Calcium ions, which play a critical role in the contraction process, are thought to be particularly important. Disturbance of Ca^{2+} transport leads to increased cytosolic Ca^{2+} which in turn further increases the ATP breakdown initiated by hypoxia. Calcium overload ultimately leads to cell death. Histologically, the dead myofibres have homogeneously eosinophilic cytoplasm (hyaline necrosis) and shrunken or fragmented nuclei. The subsequent inflammatory infiltrate consists mainly of macrophages. The lesion ultimately heals by fibrosis since cardiac muscle does not regenerate.

Cytotoxic injury is often chronic in contrast to the acute lesion caused by vasodilators. The toxic effects of antineoplastic anthracycline antibiotics such as daunorubicin and doxorubicin often appear several months after the start of therapy. The clinical picture is generally a chronic congestive cardiomyopathy. Morphologically, the two main features are cardiac dilatation and myofibre degeneration. The degeneration consists of myofibrillar loss, producing lightly stained cells, and vacuolation due to massive dilatation of the sarcoplasmic reticulum. At the ultrastructural level, many cellular components are affected. A similar chronic dose-related cardiomyopathy with congestive failure can be produced in animal models, and in rabbits the lesions tend to be distributed around blood vessels. The pathogenesis of the anthracycline cardiomyopathy is obscure. These agents have complex biochemical effects on the myocardium. These include DNA binding, inhibition of Na^+, K^+-ATPase, inhibition of coenzyme Q10-containing enzymes and promotion of lipid peroxidation. The relative importance of these biochemical changes in the initiation of chronic cardiomyopathy is unknown.

Chronic cardiomyopathies can be produced by cobalt and brominated vegetable oils. Cobalt-induced cardiomyopathy was first discovered among heavy beer drinkers in Canada. Vacuolation, swelling, loss of myofibrils and necrosis occur in experimentally poisoned rats and are found mainly in the left ventricle. Cobalt ions can complex with a variety of biologically important molecules and the potential sites for toxicity are numerous. The pathogenesis of the lesion is therefore difficult to define, but inhibition of the Krebs citric acid cycle may play an important role in an energy-dependent tissue such as the heart.

The cardiotoxicity of brominated vegetable oils is not characterised by necrosis, but by fat accumulation affecting the whole myocardium. Focal necrosis may occur in the more severely affected hearts. The heart of rats treated with brominated cottonseed oil shows a dose-related reduction in the ability to metabolise palmitic acid. This probably accounts for the accumulation of lipid globules in the myofibres.

Cardiac hypertrophy

An increase in the mass of heart muscle is occasionally found in toxicity studies. This is usually a compensatory response to an increase in workload of the heart, and in drug-related cases this is usually secondary to effects on the peripheral vasculature. Primary cardiac effects are rare, but can be produced by hormones such as growth hormones.

Cardiac pigment

Pigment deposits in the heart are a common feature of ageing animals. These ageing pigments occur in lysosomes in the perinuclear regions of the sarcoplasm, and in extensive cases the heart appears brown at necropsy. This condition is known as brown atrophy. Food colouring pigment such as Brown FK may also accumulate in a similar manner and in routine HE sections is impossible to differentiate from the lipofuscin of ageing animals.

Blood vessels

Chemically induced lesions in blood vessels are uncommon except for local reactions to intravenous injections. Systemic effects generally affect the smaller muscular arteries and arterioles and the various lesions encountered are encompassed by the general diagnosis of arteriopathy.

Arteriopathy

There are several ways to produce arteriopathy, but the lesions generally follow a similar course. In acute lesions the initial change is hyaline or fibrinoid degeneration of the intima and media. The increased eosinophilia seen histologically may be due to insudation of plasma proteins or necrosis of medial smooth muscle cells or both. An inflammatory response often ensues and the lesion may be described as an acute arteritis. Repair of the lesion is by proliferation of medial myofibroblasts extending into the intima (Figure 3.42).

The two best known pathways of vascular injury are haemodynamic changes and immune-complex deposition. Acute arterial injury can result from rapid marked haemodynamic changes produced by the exaggerated pharmacological effects of high doses of vasoactive agents. The bronchodilators and vasodilators producing cardiac necrosis may also cause an arteritis in the dog heart often in the right atrium. Agents producing vasoconstriction or hypertension such as

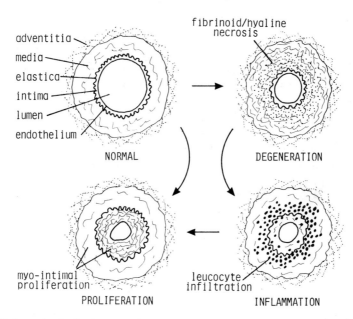

Figure 3.42. Stages in the development of arteriopathy.

noradrenaline or angiotension infusion also produce lesions in small arteries in various regions of the body. Lesions also follow alternating doses of vasodilators and vasoconstrictors. The evidence suggests that a combination of plasma leakage due to physical effects on endothelial cells and acute functional demands on the smooth muscle cell play an important role in the pathogenesis of these acute lesions.

Immune-complex lesions (vasculitis, hypersensitivity angitis) have similar features to haemodynamic lesions but tend to favour small vessels, and fibrinoid change may be less conspicuous. In animals, the lesions are produced most readily by repeated injection of foreign serum proteins. Similar 'serum sickness' lesions have occurred in man, but vasculitis has also been reported in association with drugs such as sulphonamides, quinidine and procainamide.

Arteriopathies dominated by the proliferative component have been reported in women taking oral contraceptives. The lesions consist mainly of fibromuscular intimal thickenings with little or no necrosis or leucocyte infiltrations. Vascular lesions can be produced in mice chronically dosed with steroid hormones. Intimal proliferation, sometimes leading to occlusion of the lumen, has also been reported with methysergide maleate. Finally, an arteriopathy favouring the pulmonary vessels can be produced in rats by monocrotaline, a toxic alkaloid derived from *Crotalaria spectabilis*. In chronic cases, the increased medial thickness of pulmonary arteries may produce pulmonary hypertension and right ventricular hypertrophy.

Haemorrhage

Blood may escape from vessels because of defects in clotting factors, platelets or the vessel wall, either singly or in combination. Clotting factor and platelet defects lead to haemorrhage by preventing effective closure of an injured vessel. Haemorrhage due to direct injury of the vessel wall by chemicals is infrequent except as a local toxic effect. The most common form of chemically induced haemorrhage is the widespread minor leakages that sometimes occur in the skin and mucous membranes in association with allergic vasculitis. This condition is known as purpura.

Haemorrhage is also a common artefact in animals that are dying (agonal artefact), or as a consequence of post-mortem techniques. Haemorrhage in the germinal centres of the mandibular lymph node and thymic medulla are frequent in rats killed by intraperitoneal injection of barbiturates. These haemorrhages appear as red spots on the surface of the organ. Large areas of haemorrhage may occur in the lung of rats killed by exposure to carbon dioxide and this may confound the interpretation of inhalation toxicity studies. Pulmonary haemorrhage may also occur in animals killed by physical means such as decapitation or cervical dislocation. Those cases are due to blood entering the airways, a process described as 'back-bleeding'. Care must be taken to distinguish these terminal or post-mortem events from true antemortem haemorrhages.

Haemopoietic tissue (Figure 3.43)

This is a complex system, any part of which may be the target of toxic insult. It consists primarily of bone marrow and cells in the circulating blood. The pathology of haematotoxicity can be reduced largely to effects on proliferating cells in the marrow and to effects on functional cells in the blood. The main responses observed are decreases in cell numbers, structural changes or functional abnormalities. Because the morphological responses are limited the main emphasis in this section will be on causal mechanisms.

Bone marrow

In contrast to the highly specialised and non-dividing neurone and cardiac myocyte, the sensitivity of the bone marrow to toxic injury is due to its high rate of cell division. The proliferating marrow cells may be injured by nutrient deficits, by immune attack or by direct cytotoxicity and the response is dysplasia, hypoplasia or aplasia depending on the nature and extent of the injury. The effect may be restricted to one cell line such as the erythroid series or all cell lines may be injured. This is reflected by changes in population ratios in marrow sections. Defective marrow production may cause secondary pathological changes in other parts of the body as a result of reduced or abnormal functioning cells in the peripheral blood. These include fatty change due to reduced oxygen carrying red cells (anaemia), increased susceptibility to infection due to leucocyte depletion

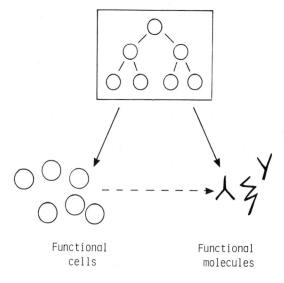

Figure 3.43. Basic organisation of the haemopoietic system.

(leucopenia) and haemorrhage as a sequel to severe platelet depletion (thrombocytopenia).

Megaloblastic change

The rapidly dividing cells of the marrow are at risk to chemicals affecting DNA synthesis and replication. Important cofactors in DNA synthesis are folates, B_{12} (cobalamin) and purine and pyrimidine nucleotides. Folates function as co-enzymes in the reduced tetrahydrofolate form, accepting and transferring one carbon fragments needed for purine and pyrimidine synthesis. Chemicals may affect either the absorption of folate from the intestine or interfere with its utilisation in the dividing cells. Chemicals interfering with absorption include diphenylhydantoin, barbiturates and ethyl alcohol. This is an example of an indirect toxic effect exerted via inhibition of essential nutrients to target cells rather than direct cytotoxicity.

Other chemicals act at the cellular level. Methotrexate inhibits folate uptake by cells, by competing for the carrier that transports reduced folate into cells. However, a more important effect is the inhibition of dihydrofolate reductase. Methotrexate impairs reduction of both folic acid and dihydrofolate thus suppressing thymidylate synthesis and subsequently DNA synthesis. In humans, megaloblastic anaemia is the classic result of inhibition of folate absorption and utilisation. The basic biochemical defect is inhibition of DNA synthesis whilst protein synthesis continues. The precursor cells are therefore unusually large (megaloblastic) before they divide. As well as being larger than the normal precursors, there is nuclear/cytoplasmic asynchrony. In megaloblastic erythrocyte precursors the apparent maturity of the cytoplasm contrasts with the immaturity of the nucleus. Giant metamyelocytes are a characteristic feature of maturation arrest in granulocyte precursors and maturation arrest of megakaryocytes may also be found. The peripheral blood picture reflects events in the marrow. The number of circulating cells is reduced and cells with abnormal structure such as macrocytic erythrocytes and hypersegmented polymorphs are evidence of abnormal maturation in the marrow.

The complete role of cobalamin co-enzymes in intermediary metabolism is less well understood. However, B_{12} is interlinked with folates in the methylation of homocysteine to methionine, a reaction that requires a cobalamin co-enzyme and 5-methyltetrahydrofolate. Lack of cobalamin leads to trapping of 5-methyltetrahydrofolate, thus depleting other folate co-enzymes used in thymidylate and DNA synthesis. The end result is megaloblastosis similar to that produced by folate deficiency. Chemicals affecting erythrocyte B_{12} metabolism act primarily by extracellular mechanisms by reducing intestinal absorption of B_{12}. They include the antituberculous drug para-aminosalicylic acid and antibiotics such as neomycin.

Megaloblastic anaemia is also a side effect of cytotoxic drugs acting via inhibition of DNA synthesis. At therapeutic doses pyrimidine antagonists such as hydroxyurea, 5-fluorouracil and cytosine arabinoside all have potent effects on DNA synthesis producing megaloblastic change. Azothioprine, 6-thioguanine and other purine antagonists also produce megaloblastic change, but less frequently than pyrimidine antagonists.

Aplasia

High doses of the potent cytotoxic drugs such as 5-fluorouracil inhibit DNA synthesis to such an extent that division virtually ceases and if the animal or patient survives, the marrow becomes aplastic. Marrow aplasia is occasionally encountered with other chemicals. Benzene produces the most reproducible effect in experimental animals, and in humans has been suggested as a cause of leukaemia in later life. A variety of other drugs and chemicals has been associated with aplasia in man but the mechanisms are unknown (idiosyncratic) and they are difficult to reproduce experimentally. One or more of the precursor populations may be affected. Chloramphenicol and phenylbutazone are two of the drugs most frequently suppressing all marrow elements resulting in pancytopenia in the peripheral blood. Chlorpromazine, thiouracil and sulphonamides tend to affect the leucocyte precursors producing a leucopenia. Chlorthiazide and quinidine occasionally cause a thrombocytopenia because of effects on platelets.

Sideroblastic anaemia

Chemicals may affect the erythrocyte series in the marrow by interfering with iron metabolism and haem synthesis. Pyridoxine (vitamin B_6) is necessary for synthesis of δ-aminolevulinic acid, a precursor of haem, and is inhibited by drugs such as the antituberculous agent isoniazid. Iron is not incorporated into haem and accumulates in mitochrondria. If the marrow is stained for iron these deposits appear as a ring around the nucleus of the normoblast and the cells are termed 'ring' sideroblasts. Lead poisoning produces a reversible sideroblastic anaemia by the inhibition of haem synthesis at several levels.

Peripheral blood

Cells circulating in the peripheral blood are susceptible to both direct and indirect chemical injury. In many cases the result is destruction or a reduced lifespan. This results in anaemia, leucopenia or thrombocytopenia depending on whether erythrocytes, leucocytes or thrombocytes are depleted. Erythrocyte destruction or a reduction in the lifespan of circulating erythrocytes is frequently termed haemolytic anaemia. Other chemicals produce functional abnormalities without any obvious structural change. The most frequent causes of injury are immune mechanisms which may affect all cell types and intracellular mechanisms which commonly affect the erythrocyte.

Immune mechanisms

These have been described mainly in man and are difficult to reproduce experimentally. Three main forms are recognised: autoimmunity, hapten-related immunity and the immune complex or 'innocent bystander' reaction. The drug α-methyldopa produces an autoimmune haemolytic anaemia in which the antibodies (predominantly IgG) are directed toward Rh determinants on the red cell surface. Red cell bound antibodies may occur in about 10% of chronically treated individuals, but less than 1% develop clinically significant haemolysis.

Hapten formation by drugs adsorbed to the cell membrane is classically associated with penicillin. The major haptenic determinant of the penicillin molecule is the benzylpenicilloyl group, and up to 3% of patients receiving large intravenous doses may develop antihapten antibodies. Fortunately, haemolytic anaemia, due to Type II immune injury, only develops in a small percentage of these. The agranulocytosis produced by aminopyrine is the neutrophil analogue of haemolytic anaemia due to hapten formation. Drugs which may attach to the surface of circulating platelets and incite antibody production include rifampicin, chlorthiazide and several sulpha drugs. A dramatic immune complex-mediated platelet destruction (Type III reaction) may occur in patients sensitised to quinine and quinidine. Circulating antibody combines with circulating drug to form an immune complex which attaches to the platelet membrane and triggers complement-mediated destruction.

Intracellular mechanisms

The number, structure and function of circulating cells may also be affected by a variety of non-immune mechanisms. Effects on red cell function are related mainly to attack on haemoglobin. The best-known example of such an agent is carbon monoxide. This competes with oxygen for the binding sites on haem to produce carboxyhaemoglobin and reduces the oxygen carrying capacity of the red cell. Other chemicals reduce oxygen-carrying capacity by oxidising the haem iron from the ferrous to the ferric state. The resultant methaemoglobin cannot combine reversibly with oxygen. Sodium nitrite, phenylhydroxylamine and other organic nitro compounds are effective oxidisers of haemoglobin. A small amount of methaemoglobin formation occurs spontaneously in red cells and the cell is equipped with reduction systems, notably methaemoglobin reductase. Methaemoglobinaemia is therefore a reversible effect.

A more severe oxidative stress may lead to oxidative haemolysis. Many of the chemicals producing this effect are aromatic compounds containing amino, nitro, or hydroxy groups. However, non-nitrogenous compounds such as chlorates also produce haemolysis and the underlying mechanisms are incompletely understood. Peroxidation may play an important role because three elements favouring peroxidation — oxygen, a transition metal ion and unsaturated lipids — are in abundant supply in the red cell. Oxidative insult can cause structural changes in haemoglobin, producing denaturation and precipitation inside the red cell. These precipitates, known as Heinz bodies, may attach to the cell membrane causing changes in permeability and possibly lysis, or deform the membrane to such an extent that cells are prematurely trapped and removed by phagocytic cells in the spleen. In addition to effects on haemoglobin, direct oxidative attack on membrane lipids may increase osmotic fragility, or alter membrane proteins and eventually lead to haemolysis.

Non-immunological effects on leucocyte numbers and function are less well studied than those on erythrocytes. Histamine, dextran and iron oxide can produce a condition known as 'pseudoneutropenia'. This is a redistribution phenomenon in which there is an increase in the marginal granulocyte pool adhering to vascular endothelium at the expense of the circulating pool, but with no net change in the total blood granulocyte pool. Conversely epinephrine can cause a rapid increase in the number of circulating granulocytes by demargination. In addition to effects on neutrophil adherence, chemicals may affect other neutrophil functions such as chemotaxis, phagocytosis, lysosomal degranulation and microbial killing. However, most of the effects are more readily demonstrated *in vitro* than *in vivo*. For example, several anti-inflammatory agents are inhibitors of chemotaxis, and colchicine and related substances will inhibit chemotaxis by their effects on microtubules. Elevated levels of galactose and glucose inhibit phagocytosis, and degranulation of lysosomes into the extracellular environment is inhibited by corticosteroids and chloroquine. Finally ethanol has multiple inhibitory effects on the neutrophil, diminishing adherence, chemotaxis and phagocytosis.

Some chemicals affect the functions of circulating platelets. Platelets are important in the arrest of bleeding following vascular disruption. They plug the wound and release factors assisting vasoconstriction and coagulation. Chemicals may affect the ability of platelets to adhere and aggregate or to release their granular constituents. Some chemicals act on the surface membrane of the platelet. For example, dipyramidole inhibits adhesion, and the antibiotic carbenicillin impairs aggregation. Other chemicals act intracellularly. Chloroquine accumulates in the serotonin granules, and aspirin irreversibly acetylates platelet cyclo-oxygenase resulting in a failure to synthesise cyclic endoperoxides and thromboxane A_2 which is a potent platelet aggregator and vasoconstrictor.

Bibliography

Skin and eye

Adams, R. M. (1983) *Occupational Skin Disease.* (New York: Grune and Stratton)
Drill, V. A. and Lazar, P. (eds.) (1980) *Current Concepts in Cutaneous Toxicity.* (New York: Academic Press)
Drill, V. A. and Lazar, P. (eds.) (1984) *Cutaneous Toxicology.* (New York: Raven Press)
Kligman, A. M. (1978) Cutaneous toxicology: an overview from the underside. *Curr. Probl. Dermatol.*, 7: 1.
Kligman, A. M. and Leyden, J. (eds.) (1982) *Assessment of Safety and Efficacy of Topical Drugs and Cosmetics.* (New York: Grune and Stratton)
Maibach, H. I. (ed.) (1975) *Animal Models in Dermatology.* (Edinburgh: Churchill Livingstone)
Marzulli, F. N. and Maibach, H. I. (eds.) (1983) *Dermatotoxicology.* (New York: Wiley)
Maurer, T. (1983) *Contact and Photocontact Allergens. A Manual of Predictive Test Methods.* (New York: Marcel Dekker)
Morris, W. E. and Kwan, S. C. (1983) Use of the rabbit ear model in evaluating the comedogenic potential of cosmetic ingredients. *J. Soc. Cosmet. Chem.*, 34: 215.
Swanston, D. W. (1983) Eye irritancy testing. In *Animals and Alternatives in Toxicity Testing*, edited by M. Balls, R. J. Riddell and A. N. Worden (London: Academic Press)

Respiratory tract

Boyd, M. R. (1980) Biochemical mechamisms in chemical induced lung injury: Roles of metabolic activation. *CRC Crit. Rev. Toxicol.*, 7: 103.
Cobb, L. M. (1981) Pulmonary toxicity. In *Testing for Toxicity*, edited by J. W. Gorrod (London: Taylor & Francis)
Hayes, J. A. (1983) Inhalational toxicology. In *A Guide to General Toxicology*, edited by F. Homburger, J. A. Hayes and E. W. Pelikan (Basel: Karger)
Menzel, D. B. and McClellan, R. O. (1980) Toxic responses of the respiratory system. In *Casarett and Doull's Toxicology, The Basic Science of Poisons*, edited by J. Doull, C. D. Klaassen and M. O. Amdur (New York: Macmillan)
Reasor, M. J., Heyneman, C. A. and Walker, C. R. (1982) Chlorcyclizine induced pulmonary phospholipidosis in rats. *Res. Comm. Chem. Pathol. Pharmacol.*, 38: 235.
Smith, A. C. and Boyd, M. R. (1983) Drug-induced pulmonary toxicity. *Trends Pharmacol. Sci.*, 4: 275.
Witschi, H. and Nettesheim, P. (eds.) (1982) *Mechanisms in Respiratory Toxicology.* (Boca Raton: CRC Press)

Gastrointestinal tract

Allen, A., Flemstrom, G., Garner, A., Silen, W. and Turnberg, L. A. (eds.) (1984) *Mechanisms of Mucosal Protection in the Upper Gastrointestinal Tract*. (New York: Raven Press)

Harmon, J. W. (ed.) (1981) *Basic Mechanisms of Gastrointestinal Mucosal Cell Injury and Protection*. (Baltimore: Williams and Wilkins)

Leegwater, D. C., De Groot, A. P. and Van Kalmthout-Kuyper, M. (1974) The aetiology of caecal enlargement in the rat. *Fd. Cosmet. Toxicol.*, 12: 687.

Pfeiffer, C. J. (ed.) (1982) *Drugs and Peptic Ulcer*, Vol. 1 and 2. (Boca Raton: CRC Press)

Rainsford, K. D. (1977) Gastrointestinal and other side-effects from the use of aspirin and related drugs: biochemical studies on the mechanisms of gastrotoxicity. *Agents Actions*, Suppl. 1: 59.

Schiller, C. M. (ed.) (1984) *Intestinal Toxicology*. (New York: Raven Press)

Visscher, G. E., Robison, R. L. and Hartman, H. A. (1980) Chemically induced lipidosis of the small intestinal villi in the rat. *Toxicol. Appl. Pharmacol.*, 55: 535.

Liver

Boyer, J. L. (1983) Mechanisms of bile formation and cholestasis. *Scand. J. Gastroenterol.*, 18 (Suppl. 87): 51.

Davis, M., Tredger, J. M. and Williams, R. (1981) *Drug Reactions and the Liver*. (London: Pitman Medical)

Farber, E. and Fisher, M. M. (1980) *Toxic Injury of the Liver*. (New York: Marcel Dekker)

Klaassen, C. D. and Watkins, J. B. (1984) Mechanisms of bile formation, hepatic uptake, and biliary excretion. *Pharmacol. Rev.*, 36: 1.

Kulkarni, A. P. and Hodgson, E. (1980) Hepatotoxicity. In *Introduction to Biochemical Toxicology*, edited by E. Hodgson and F. E. Guthrie (New York: Elsevier-North Holland)

Plaa, G. L. (1980) Toxic responses of the liver. In *Casarett and Doull's Toxicology, The Basic Science of Poisons*, edited by J. Doull, C. D. Klaassen and M. O. Amdur, (New York: Macmillan)

Plaa, G. L. and Hewitt, W. R. (eds.) (1982) *Toxicology of the Liver*. (New York: Raven Press)

Plaa, G. L. and Hewitt, W. R. (1982) Detection and evaluation of chemically induced liver injury. In *Principles and Methods of Toxicology*, edited by W. A. Hayes (New York: Raven Press)

Popper, H. (1982) Hepatocellular degeneration and death. In *The Liver, Biology and Pathobiology*, edited by A. Arias, H. Popper, D. Schachter and D. A. Shafritz (New York: Raven Press)

Schulte-Hermann, R. (1979) Reactions of the liver to injury: adaptation. In *Toxic Injury of the Liver*, edited by E. Farber and M. M. Fisher (New York: Marcel Dekker)

Slater, T. F. (1978) *Biochemical Mechanisms of Liver Injury*. (London: Academic Press)

Smuckler, E. A. (1976) Structural and functional changes in acute liver injury. *Environ. Health Perspect.*, 15: 13.

Timbrell, J. A. (1983) Drug hepatotoxicity. *Brit. J. Clin. Pharmacol.*, 15: 3.

Zimmerman, H. J. (1978) *Hepatotoxicity. The Adverse Effects of Drugs and other Chemicals on the Liver*. (New York: Appleton Century Crofts)

Kidney

Bach, P. H., Bonner, F. W., Bridges, J. W. and Lock, E. A. (eds.) (1982) *Nephrotoxicity Assessment and Pathogenesis*. (Chichester: Wiley)

Hook, J. B., McCormack, K. M. and Kluwe, W. M. (1979) Biochemical mechanisms of nephrotoxicity. In *Reviews in Biochemical Toxicology*, Vol. 1, edited by E. Hodgson, J. R. Bend and R. M. Philpot (New York: Elsevier-North Holland)

Hook, J. B. (1980) Toxic responses of the kidney. In *Casarett and Doull's Toxicology, The Basic Science of Poisons*, edited by J. Doull, C. D. Klaassen and M. O. Amdur (New York: Macmillan)

Hook, J. B. (ed.) (1981) *Toxicology of the Kidney*. (New York: Raven Press)

Porter, G. A. (ed.) (1982) *Nephrotoxic Mechanisms of Drugs and Environmental Toxins.* (New York Plenum Press)

Prescott, L. F. (1982) Assessment of nephrotoxicity. *Brit. J. Clin. Pharmacol.*, 13: 303.

Price, R. G. (1982) Urinary enzymes, nephrotoxicity and renal disease. *Toxicology*, 23: 99.

Seale, T. W. and Rennert, O. M. (1982) Mechanisms of antibiotic-induced nephrotoxicity. *Ann. Clin. Lab. Sci.*, 12: 1.

Solez, K., Racusen, L. C. and Olsen, S. (1983) The pathology of drug nephrotoxicity. *J. Clin. Pharmacol.*, 23: 484.

Solez, K. and Whelton, A. (eds.) (1984) *Acute Renal Failure. Correlations between Morphology and Function.* (New York: Marcel Dekker)

Nervous system

Astbury, P. G. and Read, N. G. (1982) Kanamycin-induced ototoxicity in the laboratory rat — a comparative morphological and audiometric study. *Arch. Toxicol.*, 50: 267.

Bron, A. J. (1979) Mechanisms of ocular toxicity. In *Drug Toxicity*, edited by J. W. Gorrod (London: Taylor & Francis).

Brummett, R. E. (1980) Drug-induced ototoxicity. *Drugs*, 19: 412.

Cavanagh, J. B. (1973) Peripheral neuropathy caused by chemical agents. *CRC Crit. Rev. Toxicol.*, 2: 365.

Davison, A. N. and Thompson, R. H. S. (eds.) (1982) *The Molecular Basis of Neuropathology*. (London: Edward Arnold)

Dewar, A. J. (1983) Neurotoxicity. In *Animals and Alternatives in Toxicity Testing*, edited by M. Balls, R. J. Riddell and A. N. Worden (London: Academic Press)

Harpur, E. S. (1981) Ototoxicological testing. In *Testing for Toxicity*, edited by J. W. Gorrod. (London: Taylor & Francis), p.219.

Jobe, P. C. and Brown, R. D. (1980) Auditory pharmacology. *Trends Pharm. Sci.*, 1: 202.

Leech, R. W. and Shuman, R. M. (1982) *Neuropathology: A Summary for Students*. (Philadelphia: Harper and Row)

McCaa, C. S. (1982) The eye and visual nervous system: anatomy, physiology and toxicology. *Environ. Health Perspect.*, 44: 1.

Mailman, R. B. (1980) Biochemical toxicology of the central nervous system. In *Introduction to Biochemical Toxicology*, edited by E. Hodgson and F. E. Guthrie (New York: Elsevier-North Holland)

Mitchell, C. L. (ed.) (1984) *Nervous System Toxicology*. (New York: Raven Press)

Norton, S. (1980) Toxic responses of the central nervous system. In *Casarett and Doull's Toxicology, The Basic Science of Poisons*, edited by J. Doull, C. D. Klaassen and M. O. Amdur (New York: Macmillan)

O'Donoghue, J. L. (1983) Neurotoxicology. In *A Guide to General Toxicology*, edited by F. Homburger, J. A. Hayes and E. W. Pelikan (Basel: Karger)

Spencer, P. S. and Schaumburg, H. H. (1980) *Experimental and Clinical Neurotoxicology*. (Baltimore: Williams and Wilkins)

Cardiovascular system

Balazs, T. (ed.) (1981/1982) *Cardiac Toxicology*, Vols. 1 and 2 (Boca Raton: CRC Press)

Balazs, T. and Ferrans, V. J. (1978) Cardiac lesions induced by chemicals. *Environ. Health Perspect.*, 26: 181.

Opie, L. H. (1980) Metabolic and drug-induced injury to the myocardium. In *Drug-Induced*

Heart Disease, edited by M. R. Bristow. (Amsterdam: Elsevier-North Holland)

Van Stee, E. W. (1978) Introduction: target organ meeting on the cardiovascular system. *Environ. Health Perspect.*, 26: 149.

Van Stee, E. W. (ed.) (1982) *Cardiovascular Toxicology.* (New York: Raven Press)

Haemopoietic tissue

Girdwood, R. H. (1979) The effects of drugs and their metabolites on blood and blood-forming organs. In *Drug Toxicity*, edited by J. W. Gorrod (London: Taylor & Francis).

Gordon-Smith, E. C. (1983) Immune drug-induced blood dyscrasias. In *Immunotoxicology*, edited by G. G. Gibson, R. Hubbard and D. V. Parke (London: Academic Press)

Hackett, T., Kelton, J. G. and Powers, P. (1982) Drug-induced platelet destruction. *Semin. Thromb. Haem.*, 8: 116.

Malpass, T. W. and Harker, L. A. (1980) Acquired disorders of platelet function. *Semin. Haematol.*, 17: 242.

Marsh, J. C. (1981) Chemical toxicity of the granulocyte. *Environ. Health Perspect.*, 39: 71.

Pisciotta, A. V. (1982) Drug-induced agranulocytosis. *Haematologica*, 67: 292.

Roncaglioni, M. C., De Gaetano, G. and Donati, M. B. (1982) Some aspects of haematological toxicity in animals. In *Animals in Toxicological Research*, edited by I. Bartosek, A. Guaitani and E. Pacei (New York: Raven Press)

Smith, R. P. (1980) Toxic responses of the blood. In *Casarett and Doull's Toxicology, The Basic Science of Poisons*, edited by J. Doull, C. D. Klaassen and M. O. Amdur (New York: Macmillan)

Swanson, M. and Cook, R. (1977) *Drugs Chemicals and Blood Dyscrasias.* (Hamilton: Drug Intelligence Publications)

4. Laboratory animal pathology

The background pathology of laboratory animals is an important confounding factor in the assessment of the toxic effects of chemicals *in vivo*. Spontaneous lesions may mimic or mask the effects of toxins and the research and regulatory toxicologists should be aware of the frequent and important lesions that occur in the commonly used species. However, a full systematic approach to laboratory animal pathology by species, by organ and by causal agent is clearly impossible in one chapter. Also toxicologists could find such a systematic approach difficult to follow or difficult to apply to the type of experimental work in which they are involved. Instead, the pathology is described in the form of the pattern of lesions that may occur in control groups of animals.

The patterns described are those seen in regulatory toxicity studies in which large numbers of tissues (Table 4.1) from large numbers of animals are examined routinely. Such studies fall into two main groups: those up to 1 year's duration in which the animals are relatively young and healthy; and chronic studies in which the animals live for the majority of their lifespan. Rat, dog and monkey are the usual species of choice in short-term studies and rat and mouse are commonly used in long-term chronic studies. The five patterns of background pathology most frequently encountered by toxicological pathologists are therefore the young rat, dog and monkey and the ageing rat and mouse. The precise details in each pattern of pathology obviously varies between laboratories depending on a variety of factors such as source and strain of animal or diet. However, there is a general theme underlying each pattern related to the incidence of lesions, the nature of these lesions, their significance to the well-being of the animal and their causes. This underlying theme will be illustrated using data from a 'typical laboratory', but the basic principles generally apply to other laboratories even though their databases may differ in detail.

As each pattern is reviewed, three aspects are highlighted: incidence of lesions, biological significance of lesions and lesions that may confound data interpretation. For example, the incidence of lesions ranges from rare to common. The biological significance of a lesion to the well-being of the animal ranges from trivial to lethal and this is at least as important in risk assessment as the incidence of lesions. Lesions cause problems in data interpretation because they mask or mimic toxic effects, or because they are difficult to classify. Distinguishing hyperplasia from neoplasia is the best-known example of the latter problem. Finally, within the context of cause-effect relationships, the young animals are described from a causation viewpoint since exogenous agents are a common cause of tissue injury. In older animals, causation is complex and includes non-specific 'ageing processes'. The pathology of the ageing rat and mouse is therefore approached on the basis of effects such as degenerations, inflammations and proliferations with particular reference to those likely to cause illness or death.

Table 4.1.   Tissues commonly examined histologically in regulatory toxicity studies.

Adrenal	Liver	Seminal vesicle
Aorta	Lung	Skeletal muscle
Bone marrow	Mandibular lymph nodes	Skin
Brain	Mesenteric lymph nodes	Spinal cord
Caecum	Mammary gland	Spleen
Colon	Oesophagus	Stomach
Duodenum	Optic nerve	Testis
Epididymis	Ovary	Thymus
Eye	Pancreas	Thyroid
Gall bladder	Parathyroid	Tongue
Heart	Pituitary	Trachea
Ileum	Prostate	Urinary bladder
Jejunum	Salivary gland	Uterus
Kidney	Sciatic nerve	Gross lesions

The young rat

The rat is the most commonly used laboratory mammal and many different strains are available, each with its own pattern of background pathology. The 'Sprague-Dawley rat' is the general reference point in this section, but even within this strain there are numerous substrains, and patterns of pathology may vary from laboratory to laboratory depending on a multiplicity of factors. This variation is largely ignored as the aim of this chapter is to review the range of pathology that may occur in rats from modern breeding colonies. One strain is used as an example, but most of the principles illustrated can be applied to pathology data from other strains in other laboratories.

Control rats rarely die in short-term studies and neoplasia is also rare. The observed pattern of pathology is therefore of non-neoplastic lesions and is usually presented in tabular form such as in Table 4.2. Only lesions occurring with an incidence greater than 1% are listed. A toxicologist presented with such a table should try to understand what the diagnoses and their frequencies mean in terms of the general background of pathology in his control animals. The first point of note is that of the 40 organs commonly evaluated only a minority have lesions, and relatively few lesions have incidence rates greater than 10%. Thus, the majority of organs of a young rat are either normal or rarely show histopathological changes. There are numerous subpatterns within this general overall pattern of infrequent lesions. The observations presented in incidence summary tables such as Table 4.2 are usually listed on an organ-by-organ basis, but lesions within any particular organ may represent degenerations, inflammations or proliferations, they may be trivial or severe and they may be related to a variety of causes. It is the association between cause and effect that is the main interest in toxicological pathology and, in young animals it is convenient to describe the pathology in terms of causation rather than in terms of lesions within any one organ. The observations in Table 4.2 can be regrouped into five major patterns of causal circumstances:

(1) Related to husbandry.
(2) Related to experimental procedures.
(3) Developmental anomalies.
(4) Miscellaneous degenerations, inflammations and proliferations.
(5) Infections and infestations.

Husbandry related

Rats are commonly housed in small groups, often in metal cages with wire mesh floors. A variety of minor external inflammatory lesions are encountered due to attrition between rats and between rats and their cages. Fur loss and dermatitis are typical changes seen on the skin and on the tail in group-housed rats. Lesions on the feet and ears may also be seen. These lesions are usually dismissed as insignificant, but differences between control and treated groups may occur in certain circumstances such as a decrease in incidence of fight wounds in rats given tranquillisers.

Procedure related

Some lesions are associated with the method of administration of the chemical or with the removal of blood samples for analysis. Rats may struggle when gavaged and the oesophagus bruised by the cannula. This bruising appears histologically as a focal myositis at any stage from an acute inflammatory to a healing lesion. The usual appearance is one of basophilic regenerating myofibres accompanied by a few leucocytes. Although the oral route is the most common method of test article administration, equivalent inflammatory lesions such as phlebitis or

Table 4.2. Example of a pattern of pathology in young rats.

Organ	Diagnosis	Percent incidence	
		Male	Female
Skin subcutis	Alopecia/fur loss	5	9
	Dermatitis/sore	4	4
Tail	Dermatitis/sore	5	3
	Other lesions	3	3
Oesophagus	Myositis	2	6
Eye	Periorbititis	10	11
	Other lesions	6	8
Heart	Leucocyte foci	7	2
Kidney	Leucocyte foci	12	7
	Hyaline droplets	15	0
	Tubular regeneration	32	4
	Mineralisation	0	6
	Hydronephrosis	10	10
Liver	Leucocyte foci	80	80
Lung	Leucocyte foci	52	56
	Pneumonitis	20	18
	Foamy histiocytes	20	16
	Mandibular lymph node		
	Hyperplasia	40	26
	Large intestine		
	Nematodes	8	3
Pituitary	Cyst	3	3
Thyroid	Ectopic thymus	2	3
Prostate	Leucocyte foci	14	—
Testis	Atrophy	2	—
Uterus	Distension	—	14

myositis may be common following intravenous and intramuscular administrations. Another lesion sometimes associated with intravenous injections is hair fragments in the lung. These fragments lodge in pulmonary vessels as hair emboli after their introduction into a peripheral vein during venepuncture. Blood sampling by orbital sinus puncture is another common procedure and this may cause a variety of inflammatory changes around the eye and orbit designated by the general term periorbitis. Repeated sampling or poor technique may produce other lesions such as degeneration of the optic nerve (optic neuropathy). The severity and incidence of these procedure-related lesions are very variable depending on the nature and frequency of the procedure and on the skill of the technician. Lesions may be uncommon and minor in short, well-conducted studies, or at the other extreme may be fatal if the oesophagus or eyeball is accidentally punctured.

Developmental anomalies

In theory, the pre- and postnatal development of any organ may be abnormal, and the severity can range from trivial to lethal. In practice, most species have well recognised groups of frequent minor anomalies equivalent to the common variants of the teratologist. Anomalies listed in Table 4.2 are pituitary cyst, ectopic thymus in thyroid, and hydronephrosis in the kidney (Figure 4.1).

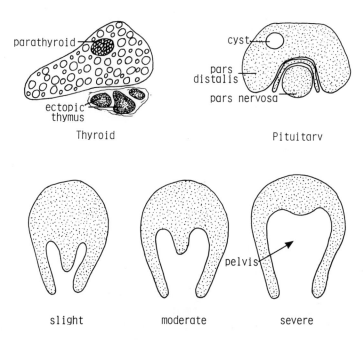

Figure 4.1. Some developmental anomalies in the young rat.

The thymus has the same embryological origin as the parathyroid and during its migration toward the base of the heart, small nests of tissue descending from the fourth branchial pouch may remain adjacent to or be embedded in the parathyroid/thyroid. These may be quite striking histologically, but are of trivial significance. Similarly, pituitary cysts are usually trivial. They are derived from remnants of the upgrowth of the craniopharyngeal (Rathke's) pouch which develops into the adenohypophysis. They vary in site and appearance, but are usually seen in the pars distalis as small colloid-filled cysts lined by ciliated epithelium. Hydronephrosis (a dilated renal pelvis) may be caused by urinary tract obstruction, but when seen as a frequent finding in control rats is usually considered a developmental or congenital anomaly. It tends to be unilateral and is usually low grade and of little significance. Severe bilateral and fatal cases may occasionally occur, but care must be taken to exclude obstruction of the lower urinary tract in these instances.

Miscellaneous pathology

A variety of minor inflammations, degenerations and proliferations of diverse or uncertain cause may be encountered in the young rat. They are grouped together as miscellaneous 'background' changes. In Table 4.2 lesions are hyaline droplets, tubular regeneration and mineralisation in the kidney, foamy histiocytes in the lung, testicular atrophy and uterine distension.

Renal hyaline droplets

These are common findings in the kidneys of males. They appear as bright eosinophilic globules of various sizes in the cytoplasm of the proximal tubular epithelium (Figure 4.2). The glomerulus of the male rat is 'leaky' to low molecular weight proteins, and these droplets represent protein resorbed by the proximal tubule cells and sequestered in lysosomes prior to recycling into the blood. Although these droplets are common and generally considered trivial, like many other background observations, the severity of the change occasionally increases in a dose-related manner. The cause of such an increase in hyaline droplets is uncertain, but may be related to interaction of the test article or a metabolite with this recycling process. In some cases, the increase in hyaline droplets is accompanied by focal tubular degeneration, which resembles the classic necrosis of compounds like mercuric chloride. Thus, a common trivial lesion may be accentuated to a sufficient extent in treated animals to be controversially interpreted as evidence of nephrotoxicity. To reiterate the importance of negative as well as positive observations in toxicology, the kidneys of females are usually normal.

Renal tubular regeneration

This is another common minor lesion in male rat kidneys. Synonyms are 'blue tubules', tubular atrophy and tubular basophilia. The affected tubules stand out against the generally eosinophilic cortex because of their basophilia. On closer inspection they appear as slightly shrunken tubules with cuboidal basophilic epithelium and sometimes a thickened basement membrane (Figure 4.2). The response of tissues to injury is limited, and tubular regeneration is one sequel to nephrotoxicity. This common trivial lesion may therefore assume importance if it confounds the interpretation of no-effect levels in studies of nephrotoxic chemicals.

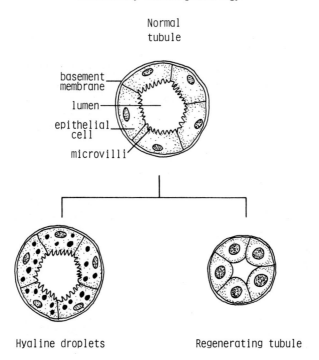

Figure 4.2. Minor renal pathology in male rats.

Renal mineralisation

Also termed nephrocalcinosis, this is a common minor renal lesion, but in this case is seen mainly in females. The mineral may be found under or in the pelvic epithelium, or more commonly in the tubules at the corticomedullary junction (Figure 4.3). The corticomedullary mineralisation usually appears between weaning and sexual maturity and the aetiology appears to be multifactorial involving dietary factors and hormones. Manipulation of dietary components in nutritional studies on certain food or protein substitutes may increase the incidence and severity of mineralisation. This is another example of interaction or synergism between the specific substance of interest and background 'factors' and it may be difficult to establish no-effect levels if there is a high incidence of mineralisation in controls.

Foamy histiocytes

In the lung, the main observation of interest is foamy histiocytes. These are also called foam cells or termed lipidosis. The condition is characterised by accumulations of plump pale cells in the alveolar lumen, often located subpleurally so that they appear at necropsy as pinpoint grey spots on the surface of the lung (Figure 4.4). The foamy appearance of these alveolar macrophages is due to the uptake

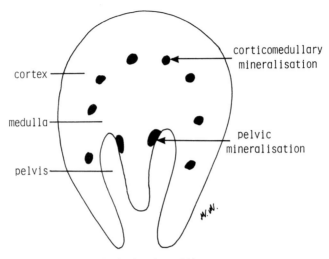

Figure 4.3. Sites of mineralisation in the female rat kidney.

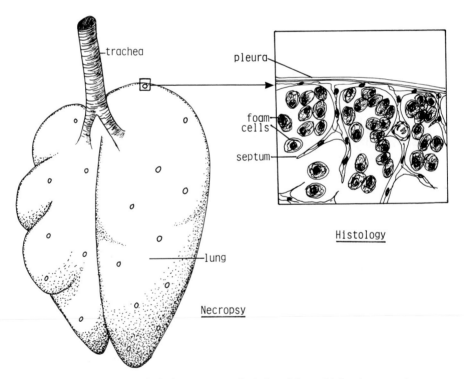

Figure 4.4. Gross and histological appearance of subpleural foamy histiocyte aggregates.

of surfactant released from Type II alveolar cells. This condition may be considered an uptake, storage and recycling process analogous to the hyaline droplets seen in the male rat kidney and, similarly, may become enhanced in response to certain treatments. This enhancement is seen most commonly in response to inhaled particles such as silica and in association with phospholipidosis-inducing compounds such as cationic amphiphilic drugs. A high control incidence of foam cells may interfere with the assessment of no-effect levels with these compounds.

Testicular atrophy

This is usually minor, unilateral and affects the subcapsular tubules. Occasionally it may be severe and diffuse, and appear at necropsy as a small, watery, blue testis (Figure 4.5). Histologically, the affected tubules are small and show partial or complete lack of germ cells leaving only Sertoli cells. This condition can have many causes including congenital origin, obstructive lesions and physical restraint as in nose-only inhalation studies. It may also result from treatment with chemicals and hormones, and a high background incidence in controls may hinder the evaluation of these substances.

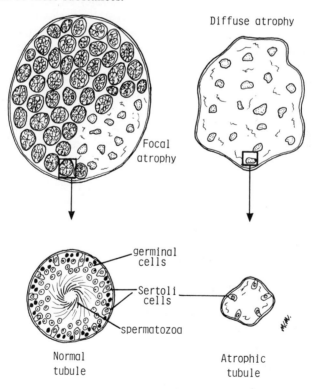

Figure 4.5. Focal and diffuse atrophy of seminiferous tubules.

Uterine distension

Distension of the uterus is not a true pathological lesion, but the pro-oestrous phase of the oestrous cycle. It may seem pointless to record this physiological variable, but some chemicals may interfere with the oestrous cycle, and the absence of distended, oedematous uteri in a large batch of animals may be the primary clue to such a response.

Leucocyte foci

These inflammatory cell foci are frequently encountered in some tissues, especially the liver and lung and to a lesser extent the prostate. They may be related to enzootic viral infections such as PVM or Sendai, but the relationship is difficult to establish. The foci are usually minor and multifocal, and usually mononuclear leucocytes in various admixtures, but mainly lymphoid. These foci appear histologically as small basophilic cellular aggregates scattered across the plane of section and are commonly recorded because they are easy to identify even at low magnifications (Figure 4.6). Other terms used are round cell foci, lymphoid foci, inflammatory foci and similar non-specific terms. This tendency to use non-specific terms is quite common amongst toxicological pathologists because of the frequent misunderstanding of the more specific terms when crossing species' lines or scientific disciplines. Thus, leucocytes in the liver may occasionally surround a necrotic liver cell and could justify the term hepatitis. However, such a diagnosis may be interpreted as a serious condition by a medical pathologist or a toxicologist unfamiliar with laboratory animal pathology. This is one of many examples where the actual choice of diagnostic terminology can significantly confound the analysis of pathology data, because different terms have different connotations of

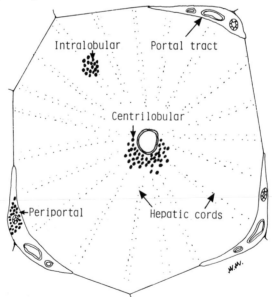

Figure 4.6. Different locations of leucocyte foci in the hepatic lobule.

biological significance to scientists with differing backgrounds.

Infections and infestations

Although many modern breeding colonies begin as caesarian-derived SPF stock, these commonly become infected at some stage in their history; or if not, the animals may become infected when transferred to toxicology units. These diseases manifest themselves in two major forms, enzootic or epizootic. Enzootic diseases are infections that are established in the colony and persist from generation to generation. They are usually stable entities which are often clinically silent and produce relatively minor pathological lesions. Epizootics on the other hand are new infections that sweep through the colony, often with obvious clinical signs and striking histological lesions. Epizootics may subsequently persist in the colony as an enzootic disease.

The pathology of infectious diseases is analogous to that of target-organ toxicity. Infectious agents may produce lesions at the site of entry equivalent to local toxicity, and lesions in the viscera equivalent to systemic toxicity. Either local or systemic effects may predominate or the disease may be manifest as a combination of both. Infectious skin disease is uncommon in most laboratory animals, and the two most frequently affected portals of entry are the respiratory and digestive tracts. In rats, infections of the respiratory tract are most frequent. Most of the remaining findings in Table 4.2 are reflections of enzootic infections.

Pinworms

These nematodes may be very common and are visible living free in the lumen of the large intestine without producing any obvious lesions. They are common in many species and are a good example of an asymptomatic local infection.

Viral pneumonitis

This is a subclinical respiratory infection. The lung lesion is a focal alveolitis that may be observed in any phase of the inflammatory process from acute to chronic and is accompanied by prominent perivascular leucocyte foci, usually lymphoid with occasional eosinophils (Figure 4.7). The alveolitis is generally of little clinical significance, but its presence can seriously confound interpretation of inhalation toxicity studies, particularly of some of the low-grade focal dust-induced lesions. Hyperplasia of the mandibular lymph node is also common in infected rats and probably represents an immune reaction to viral infection. The causal organism may be pneumonia virus of mice (PVM).

The colony used as an example in Table 4.2 was free from other enzootic or epizootic diseases at the time of sampling, but to complete this section some of the infections that may be encountered in other colonies will be briefly described.

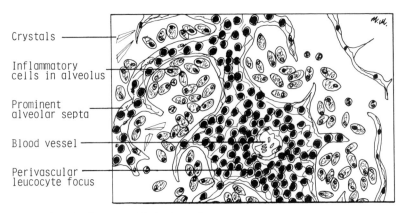

Crystals

Inflammatory
cells in alveolus

Prominent
alveolar septa

Blood vessel

Perivascular
leucocyte focus

Figure 4.7. Minor focal pneumonitis in the rat lung.

These are sialodacryoadenitis (SDA), Sendai, *Corynebacterium kutscheri* and mycoplasmal respiratory disease. These organisms cause degeneration, proliferation and inflammation in various combinations, severities and durations.

Sialodacryoadenitis

SDA is a frequent epizootic in rat colonies with a high morbidity and negligible mortality. SDA is a generic term for several serotypes of a coronavirus. These serotypes have a spectrum of virulence, primarily infecting the upper respiratory tract with variable infection of the glands around the head and neck. Respiratory tract lesions include rhinitis and focal interstitial pneumonitis, but this is generally subclinical. In contrast, infection of glands often produces striking clinical symptoms. The most striking clinical features are red staining around the eyes due to infection of the Harderian gland, and swelling of the ventral neck region associated with infection of the submaxillary salivary gland. The swollen neck, 'rat mumps', rapidly subsides and the rats appear normal within about a week. SDA is thus a disease dominated by acute local effects. The main finding at necropsy, depending on the stage of the disease, is a swollen or shrunken salivary gland. Histologically, the gland progressively shows various combinations of degeneration, inflammation and regeneration, but is quickly restored to normal (Figure 4.8). The Harderian gland shows a similar cycle of disease, but squamous metaplasia is very prominent in the proliferative repair phase.

Sendai

Sendai is a paramyxovirus which is enzootic in many modern rat colonies. Enzootic infections generally affect weanlings as maternal milk-transmitted immunity wanes. The pups develop a respiratory disease that is generally subclinical. At necropsy, many rats appear normal, but some have small red foci scattered over the surface of the lung. Histologically, there are acute necrotising inflammatory

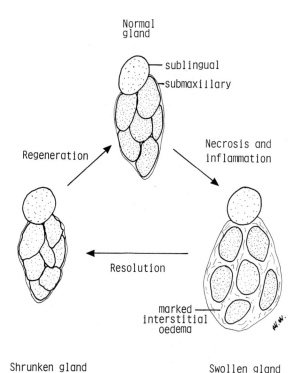

Figure 4.8. Gross appearance of SDA infection in submaxillary salivary gland.

lesions in the mucosal epithelium of the nose, trachea and pulmonary airways, the last often extending into the alveoli. Most of the airway mucosal lesions repair rapidly and completely, but focal fibrosis and scarring may occur in terminal airways and associated alveoli. In general, however, Sendai can be considered an acute transient infection of the rat respiratory tract with little or no residual effects.

Corynebacterium kutscheri

This is another example of a disease dominated mainly by acute local effects in the respiratory tract. The infection is usually latent or inapparent, but may become activated to produce acute suppurative pulmonary lesions which are either fatal, or resolve by fibrosis and the formation of granulomas (Figure 4.9). Activation of this disease is usually attributed to 'resistance lowering factors'. Administration of chemicals could be such a factor either through immunosuppression or the general stress of toxicity. A pathologist could be presented with a pattern of zero or minor lesions in controls and a dose-related increase in lung lesions in treated groups. This apparent 'pulmonary toxicity' is another example of the complex interaction between different causal agents that may occur in animal models.

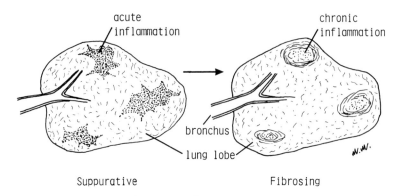

Figure 4.9. Sequence of *C. kutscheri* pneumonia.

Mycoplasmosis

The final example of an infectious disease that may be encountered is mycoplasmosis. Mycoplasmosis tends to be tissue and host specific, and in the rat the disease primarily affects the respiratory tract and to a lesser extent the female reproductive tract. In contrast to the previous acute infections it is a chronic condition and rat respiratory mycoplasmosis is commonly termed 'chronic respiratory disease'. This disease has been eliminated from most modern colonies, but is still occasionally encountered as a highly contagious, chronic enzootic disease of the respiratory tract. The most spectacular pathological changes are seen in the old rat when the lung may be converted to a mass of bronchiectatic abscesses, but the disease begins in early life. The most characteristic clinical sign in the young rat is snuffling and wheezing during the first 3 months of life. This snuffling is associated with inflammation in the upper respiratory tract, notably rhinitis, and with increasing severity or age progressively affects the larynx, trachea and lungs to produce the bronchiectatic abscess characteristic of the older rat. The histopathological finding is fairly typical of chronic disease in that it largely consists of a mixture of chronic inflammation and reparative proliferation (Figure 4.10).

After mycoplasmal colonisation small amounts of purulent exudate appear in the airway lumen. This is followed by hyperplasia and increased mucus production in the respiratory epithelium and by lymphoid infiltration and proliferation. The hallmarks of chronic infection are thus exudate, epithelial hyperplasia, squamous metaplasia and lymphoid cell accumulation. The infection may also affect the middle ear, and subsequent labrynthitis may produce clinical symptoms such as circling. Like *C. kutscheri* infection, the disease pattern may be altered by extraneous factors such as ammonia levels in the animal room as well as by interaction with other infectious agents such as Sendai and of course by effects related to test article administration.

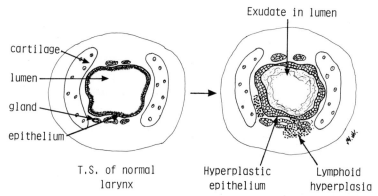

Figure 4.10. Chronic respiratory disease in the larynx. TS = Transverse section.

Summary

The young rat has been described at some length to illustrate the basic patterns of pathology that occur in young animals and also to show the way in which these patterns may confound the interpretation of data in toxicity studies. Although the causes of injury are different from the toxins described in Chapter 3, the end results — degeneration, proliferation and inflammation — are essentially the same which re-emphasises the axiom that the ways in which the body can respond to injury are limited.

In terms of the two basic scales for assessing lesions — incidence and severity — pathology findings in the young rat can be considered to be generally infrequent, and when present, of minor biological significance. Their main importance is in the two ways in which they can complicate the interpretation of treatment-related responses. In the first place they may mimic the effect of treatment. For example, renal tubular regeneration may complicate the assessment of no-effect levels of nephrotoxins. Secondly, the incidence or severity of background pathology may be enhanced in a dose-related manner. The enhancement may be of endogenous processes such as the lysosomal cycling of pulmonary surfactant and renal protein, or it may be of processes initiated by exogenous agents such as infections. In either case, the precise causal relationship of treatment to the observed response may be difficult to unravel.

The young dog

The beagle is the usual animal of choice in regulatory toxicity studies. These animals are laboratory bred, of known parentage, generally free of disease, a convenient size and easy to handle. The pattern of pathology findings in these young dogs (Table 4.3) resembles that of the young rat in that lesions are generally infrequent and usually of a minor nature. They can be grouped into the same five causal patterns.

Husbandry related

Dogs are housed in cages in some countries, but in the UK the usual practice is to house them in pens with concrete floors sprinkled with sawdust. The dogs may be housed singly, in groups, or singly with communal exercise runs. As in the rat, skin lesions related to husbandry are quite common. The two main types are abrasions due to concrete surfaces and wounds caused by fighting. Sawdust is also responsible for a few lesions, notably a dust-related conjunctivitis, and a focal granulomatous glossitis due to fragments embedded in the tongue. Some focal inflammatory lesions in the lung may also be due to inhaled sawdust, but this is difficult to establish with certainty.

Procedure related

No procedure-related lesions are listed in Table 4.3. These control data were derived from studies using the dietary or gavage route of administration and it is very unusual to find any damage due to these procedures other than the very rare case of accidental lung dosing. Similarly, removal of blood samples from the cephalic vein of the conscious animal is relatively simple and these sites are not routinely examined histologically.

Developmental anomalies

These are generally infrequent, minor and associated mainly with endocrine tissues. As in the rat, the pattern includes cysts in various organs, notably the pituitary, and ectopic thymus around the thyroid and parathyroid.

Miscellaneous pathology

A range of minor, usually focal, degenerations, inflammations and proliferations is encountered. Although these entities are easily recognised, the cause is often difficult to establish and they are grouped into the general category of miscellaneous pathology. The main entities are mineralisations, a spectrum of inflammations in various organs ranging from leucocyte foci to various forms of '-itis', C-cell hyperplasia in the thyroid, telangiectasis in the spleen and changes in the status of the reproductive tract.

Mineralisations

Minor foci of mineralisation are very common in the kidney. In contrast to the rat, these basophilic deposits are located in the renal papilla and occur in both sexes. Mineralisation in the stomach also occurs quite frequently in both sexes. The histological appearance is quite striking and usually appears as basophilic granules contrasting with the eosinophilic oxyntic cells of the middle to upper third of the fundic mucosa (Figure 4.11). Mineralisation is also found occasionally in the aortic media near the base of the heart.

Table 4.3. Example of a pattern of pathology in young beagles.

Organ	Diagnosis	Percent incidence	
		Male	Female
Skin	Sores, wounds etc.	7	4
Eye	Sores, conjunctivitis	4	4
Tongue	Glossitis	2	1
Heart	Leucocyte foci	1	1
Blood vessels	Arteritis	2	2
	Aortic mineralisation	2	3
Small intestine	Nematode	28	23
	Granuloma	4	2
Large intestine	Granuloma	1	3
Kidney	Leucocyte foci	4	1
	Mineralisation	74	69
	Interstitial nephritis	6	6
	Pyelitis	4	7
	Granuloma	0	4
Liver	Leucocyte foci	60	47
	Granuloma	4	2
Lung	Leucocyte foci	18	17
	Bronchitis/bronchiolitis	8	2
	Pneumonitis	22	28
	Fibrosing alveolitis	3	1
	Granuloma	7	6
	Nematode	2	6
Mesenteric lymph node	Granuloma	27	21
Parathyroid	Cyst	1	0
Pituitary	Cyst	24	26
Spleen	Telangiectasis	14	7
Stomach	Mineralisation	10	7
Thymus	Ectopic thyroid	1	0
	Cyst	1	1
Thyroid	Ectopic thymus	2	1
	Cyst	2	1
	C-cell hyperplasia	8	9
	Lymphoid hyperplasia	2	0
Prostate	Leucocyte foci	12	—
	Prostatitis	12	—
Testis	Focal atrophy	5	—
Uterus	Distension	—	11

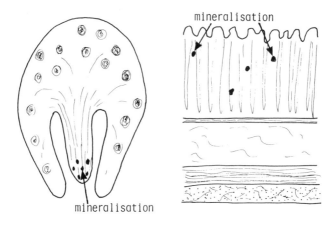

Kidney papilla   Fundic mucosa

Figure 4.11. Common mineralisations in young beagles.

Telangiectasis

Telangiectasis (dilated blood vessels) occurs in the spleen and heart valves. In the spleen it is most conspicuous in exsanguinated dogs as dark red blebs around the margin of the spleen. Histologically, these blebs consist of blood-filled sinusoids which fail to empty during the splenic contraction associated with exsanguination. This distribution is similar to that of siderotic nodules in older dogs and may well be the precursor lesion. Another, but much less frequent telangiectatic condition is valvular telangiectasis in the atrioventricular valves of the heart. This appears as small blood cysts at necropsy and as blood-filled endothelial-lined channels in histological sections.

Inflammations

Lung, liver, kidney and prostate are the organs most commonly containing minor leucocyte foci or inflammatory reactions. Inflammatory reactions in lung can be caused by agents arriving via the airways or via the bloodstream and a diverse range of minor inflammatory lesions may be encountered. These are often in different stages of the inflammatory process and it is usually difficult to define the aetiology unless the cause is obvious such as foreign body granulomas. Lesions are therefore recorded as present or absent usually without any attempt to define the aetiology. Simple foci of leucocyte accumulation, low-grade bronchitis/bronchiolitis and minor alveolar inflammations (pneumonitis) are the most frequently encountered non-specific lesions. A more specific entity but still of uncertain aetiology is fibrosing alveolitis. This appears grossly as raised white foci or plaques often on the ventral third of the anterior lobes of lung. Histologically, these lesions are subpleural wedge-shaped areas with prominent alveolar living cells and fibrotic interstitium.

    Foci of leucocyte accumulation, often around the portal tracts, are common in the liver, but other inflammatory foci are generally infrequent. Similarly, in the kidney relatively few inflammations are found other than minor focal interstitial nephritis and pyelitis. The histological appearance of interstitial nephritis is somewhat similar to tubular regeneration in the rat except that in addition to tubular distortion and basophilia, there is an interstitial accumulation of leucocytes, mainly lymphoid cells (Figure 4.12). Usually, only one or two small groups of cortical tubules are affected and use of the term 'interstitial nephritis' may cause problems in data review. Interstitial nephritis is a common disease in old dogs, often diffuse and of sufficient severity to cause death in some cases. Thus the term interstitial nephritis, like hepatitis, can be misinterpreted by reviewers who are not familiar with the background pathology of young laboratory animals. What is a trivial lesion may be mis-read as equivalent to a sub-lethal condition if the all-important qualifying terms focal and minimal are omitted or ignored. Pyelitis may have similar connotations as a severe disease, but in young beagles it is usually a localised entity of a minor nature characterised by focal infiltrations of mononuclear leucocytes into the epithelium and lamina propria of the renal pelvis. The pelvic epithelium may be slightly hyperplastic in some cases (Figure 4.12).

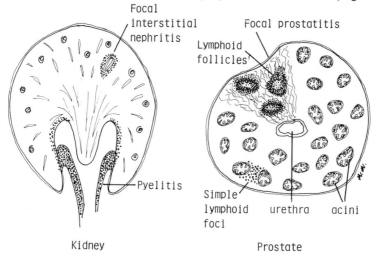

Figure 4.12. Common urogenital tract lesions in young beagles.

The other common lesion in the urogenital tract of the young dog is in the prostate. Like interstitial nephritis and pyelitis the main histological feature is lymphoid cell accumulation. This can range from minor leucocyte foci to large lymphoid aggregates with germinal centre formation. The latter may be accompanied by epithelial atrophy and interstitial fibrosis (Figure 4.12). The focal cell accumulations unaccompanied by any other changes are termed leucocyte foci as in other tissues, but the larger lesions with epithelial changes have to be termed prostatitis. Again, this is a controversial diagnosis and illustrates the importance of qualifying terms because acute prostatitis with signs of systemic illness is common in veterinary practice in the older dog whereas prostatitis as seen in young beagles is an asymptomatic focal subacute or chronic inflammatory lesion.

Lymphoid accumulations also occur occasionally in the thyroid. They may develop to the extent of germinal centre formation, but rarely cause follicle destruction. Occasionally such destruction is encountered, resulting in a histological appearance of lymphocytic thyroiditis resembling autoimmune thyroiditis in man.

The final inflammatory condition of interest is arteritis. This is sometimes encountered incidentally in the heart and in organs such as the thyroid. The usual appearance is of fibrinoid change in the media accompanied by varying degree of leucocyte accumulation in the adventitia and outer media. The aetiology is uncertain, but the affected vessels are often small-calibre branches of larger elastic arteries suggesting local pressure effects. A more widespread form of arteritis is occasionally seen in which the inflammatory reaction is very pronounced. The dogs sometimes show ill-defined clinical symptoms. The aetiology is uncertain, but is possibly an allergic vasculitis.

Hyperplasias

As might be expected, these are infrequent in the young dog. The one most frequently encountered is C-cell hyperplasia in the thyroid. The appearance of the C-cell population in the dog thyroid is extremely variable, but occasionally large, tumour-like, islands may be encountered. Although these can be designated as hyperplasias, they may equally well be developmental anomalies.

Sexual maturity

Reproductive tract pathology, other than lymphocytic prostatitis, is uncommon. However, the physiological status of the reproductive tract can be a significant confounding factor in short-term toxicity studies. Dogs are usually introduced into toxicity studies about 6–9 months of age, just before sexual maturity. During the next few weeks, some dogs may become sexually mature, and bitches may enter their first oestrous cycle. There is a vast difference in gonad weights between mature and immature animals and it is not unknown for all the late-maturing animals to be assigned purely by chance to the highest dose group. The small testes of these immature dogs could be misinterpreted as testicular atrophy. Not only may chance allocation act as a confounding factor, but late maturity may be a secondary effect of poor growth due to toxicity and result in a dose-related sexual immaturity. Because of these two variables, toxic effects on the reproductive tract in short-term studies in the dog are much more difficult to interpret than those occurring in the much more rapidly maturing rat.

Infections and infestations

These are uncommon in laboratory-bred beagles. The three main infectious problems in veterinary medicine — distemper, viral hepatitis and leptospirosis — are controlled by routine vaccination programmes, and most metazoan parasites are removed by therapeutic procedures. However, some may persist to be found in dogs used in toxicity studies.

Roundworms

Roundworms (*Toxocara canis* or *Toxascaris leonina*) often seem to persist in small numbers, and several findings in Table 4.3 relate to these organisms, notably *Toxocara canis*. This ascarid worm undergoes a tissue migratory cycle prior to establishing itself in the upper small intestine (Figure 4.13).

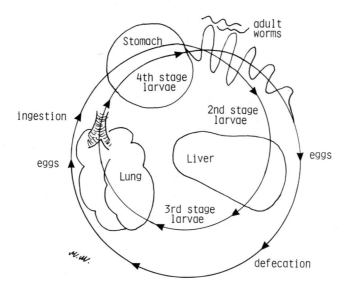

Figure 4.13. Life cycle of *Toxocara canis*.

The adults are white worms generally 4–10 cm long which live free in the gut lumen and pass eggs into the faeces. These contaminate the environment and may be ingested by other animals, including man. Second-stage larvae hatch from ingested eggs and penetrate the intestinal mucosa. The usual route of larval migration is to the liver and then via the venous blood to the lungs. Larvae leave the pulmonary vessels, moult and pass via the trachea to the intestines where they mature. Some larvae may undergo a somatic migration and reach other tissues. The pathological syndrome presented by *Toxocara canis* is thus of white adult worms in the small intestine at necropsy and gross or histological lesions in various tissues related to systemic larval migration. Dead or moulting larvae incite a granulomatous reaction with a prominent eosinophil component, and such granulomas are highly suggestive of larval migration even if the larva or dead remnants are not present. The mesenteric lymph node and lung are the most common sites of granuloma formation, but granulomas are occasionally seen in other sites such as the renal cortex. Because larval migration can occur in man, *Toxocara canis* is an important zoonotic disease and occasional cases of blindness due to migration through the retina are reported in children.

Lungworm
Another parasite occasionally seen in laboratory beagles is the lungworm (*Filaroides* sp.). This worm is usually an incidental histological observation in the lung. In contrast to *Toxocara canis* the worm often resides in the alveoli without inciting any significant inflammatory response.

Parvovirus
An epizootic disease of major clinical significance since late 1970s is canine parvovirus. This virus has an affinity for rapidly dividing tissues and causes two main disease syndromes, myocarditis in puppies and enteritis in older animals. Myocarditis occurs in puppies about 4–8 weeks old and has a high mortality rate which can decimate breeding colonies. The disease is now largely controlled by vaccination, but if there is high exposure to virulent virus, myocardial lesions may still occur in weanlings.

Summary
The pattern of pathology in the young beagle is basically similar to that encountered in the young rat. Pathology findings are generally infrequent, and when present are usually of minor biological significance. As in the rat, background pathology may confuse toxicological interpretation, but is often more difficult to unravel within the context of a single study because relatively few animals are used. An understanding of the general pattern expected in young beagles is therefore an important factor in the interpretation of toxicity studies.

The young baboon

Many types of monkey such as rhesus, cynomolgus, marmoset and baboon are used in toxicology, but they are used less frequently than the dog as a non-rodent species. Since fewer animals are used, across a wide range of species, control databases tend to be fragmentary. Several primate breeding centres have been established in various parts of the world. The most frequently used laboratory-bred animals are rhesus monkeys and marmosets. In established, well-run breeding colonies, the background pattern of pathology generally resembles that of other laboratory-bred animals, namely infrequent and minor lesions, and these need not be reiterated. However, wild-caught animals are still in common use and toxicologists need to be aware of the range of lesions that may be found in such animals. The wild-caught young baboon will be used as the reference point for this section, with occasional comment on other species. In general, monkeys undergo a considerable conditioning period at the importers before supply to the toxicology laboratory, and once in the laboratory they usually undergo a further period of conditioning. The health of these animals is therefore much better than the term 'wild-caught' might imply, and in some cases the incidence of pathology findings may be less than in the laboratory-bred beagle. In other instances, lesions may be frequent, particularly those due to metazoan parasites. Overall, however, the basic pattern is one of infrequent and generally minor lesions. Some of the more common findings are listed in Table 4.4 and discussed below.

Husbandry related
Young monkeys are usually housed individually in metal cages. Many of the husbandry-related conditions tend to be self-inflicted. Chewing and gnawing of skin is occasionally seen and may result in severe lesions. Trapped and broken limbs are occasionally encountered due to the monkey reaching through the cage bars, but these are rare events. Nutritional diseases are also rare events in modern laboratories, but were a considerable cause of morbidity and mortality in the past.

Procedure related
Lesions related to gavage are relatively rare but focal congestion of the stomach mucosa is sometimes seen. Veins are smaller than in the dog, but experienced technicians can remove blood samples with little difficulty. The most significant procedure-related lesions are injuries caused during restraint, but these should be rare in well-managed units. Probably the most common procedure-related injury is not in the monkey, but bite wounds on the technicians — even with the most skilled personnel.

Developmental anomalies
The range of developmental anomalies is similar to that in the dog and rat and associated mainly with endocrine tissues. Ectopic thymus located around the thyroid is very common and cysts are occasionally encountered in various tissues. Accessory nodules of cortical tissue are common in the adrenal capsule and occasionally occur at other sites. Ectopic bone in the adrenal is one of the more striking anomalies. The appearance ranges from a small fragment of bone to a bony nodule complete with bone marrow. Ectopic splenic tissue in the pancreas may occasionally create diagnostic problems because it resembles an inflammatory focus if the area is sectioned tangentially.

Miscellaneous pathology
Although exotic lesions are sometimes encountered, the general background of miscellaneous pathology is similar to that of other young animals, with mineralisations, leucocyte foci and various forms of '-itis' predominating. The main exception is the high incidence of pigmented histiocytes in the lung. These are perivascular aggregates of plump, light brown cells which are strikingly birefringent when examined using polarised light. These cells contain dust particles inhaled during life in the wild, and are a form of pneumoconiosis.

The state of maturity of the reproductive tract is less of a problem in young baboons than it is in dogs. The precise age of wild-caught animals is unknown, but they often have their milk teeth and the reproductive tract is immature. Most of the animals are probably 2–3 years old, and as sexual maturity is around 5–6 years of age maturation during the course of a toxicity study is uncommon.

Table 4.4. Example of a pattern of pathology in young baboons.

Organ	Diagnosis	Percent incidence Male	Female
Skin subcutis	Dermatitis	1	4
	Granuloma/abscess		2
Tongue	Granuloma	3	2
Adrenal	Steatosis	4	11
	Mineralisation	5	5
	Bone		2
Brain	Leucocyte foci	4	4
Heart	Leucocyte foci	6	4
Large intestine	Granuloma	9	14
	Nematodes	1	1
Small intestine	Granuloma	2	
	Enteritis	1	2
	Nematodes	3	1
	Tapeworm	1	
Kidney	Leucocyte foci	24	18
	Interstitial nephritis	12	9
	Mineralisation	11	7
Liver	Leucocyte foci	59	64
	Granuloma	16	10
	Abscess	2	
	Kupffer cell pigment	5	2
Lung	Leucocyte foci	7	7
	Pigmented histiocytes	68	70
	Bronchitis/bronchiolitis	3	4
	Pneumonitis	2	5
	Granuloma	1	3
Lymph node	Hyperplasia	2	2
	Pigment	1	6
	Granuloma		2
Muscle:	Sarcocyst	3	1
Pancreas	Ectopic spleen	3	5
Pituitary	Cyst	10	17
Salivary gland	Leucocyte foci	23	24
	Mineralisation		3

Spleen	Follicular hyperplasia	3	7
	Pigment	4	3
	Capsular fibrosis	4	1
Stomach	Nematodes	2	2
	Gastritis	1	2
Thymus	Cyst		3
Thyroid	Ectopic thymus	50	60
Trachea	Tracheitis	1	4
Testis	Immature	94	—
Ovary	Immature	—	87
	Mineralisation	—	40

In other wild-caught monkeys, such as cynomolgus, a batch supplied to a toxicology laboratory may contain a mixture of animals of varying sexual maturity. Care should be taken to avoid allocating mature animals to one treatment group and immature animals to another. A slightly different problem occurs in mature rhesus monkeys. These are seasonal breeders and physiological regression of the testes should not be mistaken for chemically induced atrophy.

Infections and infestations

Acute viral and bacterial epizootics, mainly affecting the lung and digestive tract, may be frequent during the pre-study conditioning period. However the animals must be clinically free of such disease symptoms before the study is allowed to start and lesions such as pneumonia and enteritis are usually infrequent during routine toxicity studies. In the conditioned animals used in toxicity studies pathology findings are dominated by parasites. Many of the lesions in Table 4.4 such as granulomas are due to parasites which may or may not be visible and identifiable. The incidence of parasite infestation varies enormously between different batches of animals depending on the region of origin, but over a period of time a wide range of protozoan and metazoan parasites may be seen. The most frequently occurring parasites are listed in Table 4.5.

Protozoa

Protozoan infections are common in baboons (Figure 4.14). *Balantidium* sp. are large ovoid ciliated amoeba-like organisms living free in the large intestine. They are usually non-pathogenic, but have been associated with cases of ulcerative enteritis. *Sarcocystis* sp. also appears to be largely non-pathogenic. This coccidian

Table 4.5.   Parasites frequently found in baboons.

PROTOZOA	TREMATODE
Balantidium sp.	*Schistosoma* sp.
Hepatocystis sp.	CESTODE
Sarcocystis sp.	*Bertiella* sp.
NEMATODE	ARTHROPOD
Abbreviata sp.	*Rhinophaga* sp.
Oesophagostomum sp.	

parasite has an obligatory two-host life cycle. Carnivores are the definitive host in which the sexual phase occurs in the small intestine. Sporulated oocytes shed in the faeces contaminate the environment and may be ingested by another host. Sporozoites invade tissues, undergo a schizogony phase and finally encyst, typically in striated muscle. The cysts are commonly encountered in the striated muscles of the limbs, diaphragm and tongue and even rarely in the heart. They do not incite any host response and appear histologically as granular basophilic bodies amongst the eosinophilic myofibres.

Hepatocystis kochi is a malarial parasite transmitted by midges. Sporozoites enter the blood via bite wounds and undergo schizogony in the liver. Schizogony in hepatocytes produces large merocysts which coalesce to produce 2–4 mm diameter white foci on the surface of the liver. Histologically, the mature cyst has a central fluid-filled space and a periphery filled with pale basophilic merozoites. There is little host reaction until the cyst degenerates or ruptures to release merozoites into the blood. The host reaction is granulomatous with a prominent eosinophil and giant-cell component ultimately leading to a fibrous scar, which sometimes shows mineralisation.

Nematodes

A wide variety of nematode species may be found in baboons, but *Abbreviata* sp. and *Oesophagostomum* sp. are among those most commonly observed to produce lesions (Figure 4.15): *Abbreviata* sp. resemble roundworms in the dog, but they are attached to the stomach mucosa producing erosions, ulcers and various degrees of gastritis.

Oesophagostomum is commonly known as the nodular worm because of the characteristic nodule produced in the large intestine. Typical nodules are 2–4 mm diameter, smooth, black-brown and easily visible on the serosal surface at necropsy. The histological appearance varies depending on the age of the nodule, but usually appears as a granulomatous encapsulation of histiocytes, eosinophils and lymphoid cells surrounding debris in which one or more cross sections of nematode are visible. In about 1 week, the nodule ruptures and the worm escapes into the lumen and matures. The residual nodule appears histologically as a focus of fibrosis and pigmented histiocytes in the wall of the large intestine. Other nematodes seen in the large intestine are pinworms (oxyurids) and whipworms

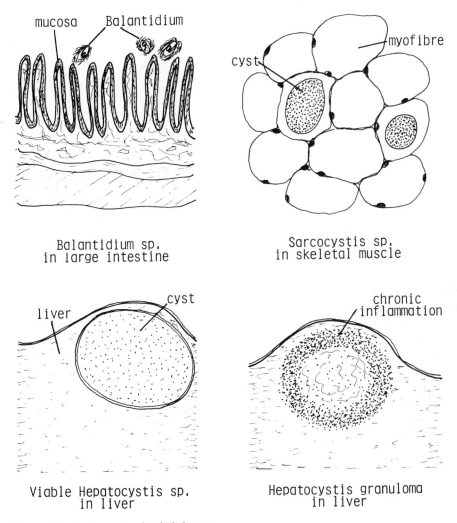

mucosa   Balantidium

cyst

myofibre

Balantidium sp.
in large intestine

Sarcocystis sp.
in skeletal muscle

liver   cyst

chronic
inflammation

Viable Hepatocystis sp.
in liver

Hepatocystis granuloma
in liver

Figure 4.14. Protozoan parasites in baboons.

(trichurids) but these live free in the lumen producing no pathological lesions under normal circumstances. In other monkeys, different nematodes may be found such as *Gongylonema* sp. which reside in the stratified squamous epithelium of the upper digestive tract and *Nochtia* sp. which incite a focal papillomatous proliferation in the stomach.

Trematodes

Schistosomiasis is the most frequently encountered trematode infection producing histological lesions. These small unisexual dimorphic flukes live in the blood. Lesions can result from adults in the veins, but the most common lesions observed

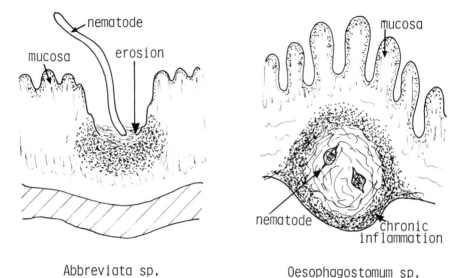

Abbreviata sp.
erosion in stomach

Oesophagostomum sp.
nodule in large intestine

Figure 4.15. Nematode lesions in baboons.

histologically are intense focal granulomatous responses to ova penetrating the wall of the small intestine or deposited in the liver (Figure 4.16). Blood may be present in the faeces of heavily infested animals. This may confound faecal occult blood tests commonly applied in toxicity tests of non-steroidal anti-inflammatory agents. Orange flukes (*Watsonius* sp.) are occasionally seen in the large intestine of baboons from West Africa, but these are not generally associated with any significant lesions. Another fluke of interest is *Paragonimus* sp. in the cynomolgus monkey. This fluke is unusual in that it resides in the lung.

Cestodes

The incidence of cestode infestations in baboons is highly variable. Infestations are usually light and not associated with any pathological lesions. However, some prosectors find the length, colour and slow contractile movements of tapeworms disturbing and this is probably their main impact in toxicological pathology. *Bertiella* sp. are the ones most frequently encountered. These can reach 0.5 m in length, but the large globular scolex has no rostellum or hooks and they are clinically insignificant.

Arthropods

Most arthropod infestations are generally associated with the skin. These ectoparasites, such as lice, are generally removed during the conditioning period and rarely observed in toxicity studies. The infestations most frequently encountered are those associated with extracutaneous sites, notably mites in the

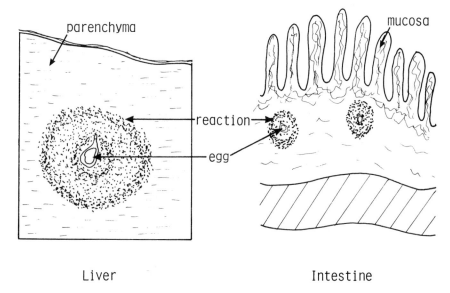

Figure 4.16. Granulomas caused by schistosome ova.

respiratory tract. The actual mite (*Rhinophaga* sp.) is rarely observed in the baboon lung, but its presence can be recognised in the larger airways by an oedematous bronchial mucosa moderately infiltrated by eosinophils (Figure 4.17). In contrast, the lung mite (*Pneumonyssus* sp.) of the rhesus monkey is commonly encountered in histological section of peripheral lung associated with a focal pneumonitis containing numerous eosinophils and accumulations of brown-black pigment.

Summary

The pattern of pathology in the young wild-caught, laboratory-conditioned baboon and other primates is essentially similar to that observed in the young rat and beagle. Pathology findings are infrequent and generally minor with a variable superimposition of lesions due to protozoan and metazoan infestations. The incidence of these parasitic lesions varies between batches of monkeys, but even in heavily parasitised animals, the lesions are usually granulomatous inflammations with a prominent eosinophil component and are unlikely to be confused with the majority of toxic responses.

The ageing rat

The pathology of the ageing rat is an important confounding factor in long-term toxicity studies used as bioassays for chronic toxicity and carcinogenicity. In contrast to the relatively simple pattern of infrequent and generally minor lesions seen in young animals the pattern seen in animals ageing during chronic studies

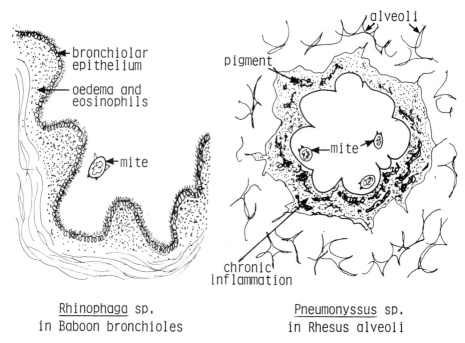

Rhinophaga sp.
in Baboon bronchioles

Pneumonyssus sp.
in Rhesus alveoli

Figure 4.17. Lung mite lesions.

is one of an increasing incidence and severity of lesions culminating in death. Although lesions related to husbandry, procedures, development and infections still occur, these are relatively minor compared with the main age-associated lesions and therefore the pattern of pathology will be classified in a different way. The three main effects of interest in chronic rodent studies are morbidity/mortality, non-neoplastic lesions and neoplasms. The general pattern of pathology in the ageing Sprague-Dawley is described in terms of these three response endpoints rather than by that of causation as used for the younger animals.

Morbidity/mortality

The two main parameters of interest in analysis of morbidity (illness) and mortality (death) are the rate at which they occur and the causation. These data give the toxicologist an excellent opportunity to overview some of the major background characteristics of the rat strain. One or both of these parameters may be affected by treatment.

Rate

The general survival pattern for one substrain of Sprague-Dawley rat housed five per cage and fed *ad libitum*, in one conventional laboratory is shown in Figure 4.18. The animals are 6–8 weeks old at the start of the study and may be removed from the study through either illness or death. The curve is thus a composite of morbidity and mortality rather than a true survival curve. The removal of sick rats is general practice in toxicity studies to avoid the loss of valuable tissues through cannibalism or autolysis. The curves vary slightly from study to study, but over 90% of animals are still on study at 78 weeks and then survival begins to decline rapidly and almost linearly. At 104 weeks, approximately 40–50% females and 60–70% of males are still alive and this is reduced to 25% at about 112 and 136 weeks respectively.

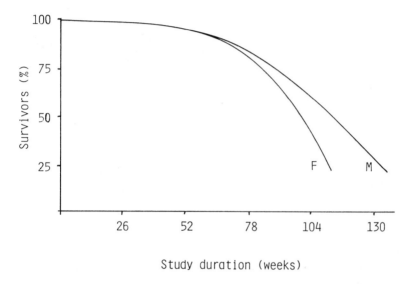

Figure 4.18. Survival curves for conventionally housed Sprague-Dawley rats, 6–8 weeks old at study initiation. F = Female; M = Male.

The rate of morbidity and mortality is an important factor in the design of long-term studies. Long-term studies are divided into two main groups, 2-year studies and lifespan studies. In 2-year studies the rats are killed at a specific point in time. In lifespan studies, the study is terminated when survival is reduced to 20–25%. Lifespan studies usually exceed 2 years' duration. The arguments for and against each choice of timescale are complex, but are essentially related to practical problems and assay sensitivity. A 2-year study is much simpler to handle logistically. Schedules and report dates are firm and the capacities of the toxicology facilities can be utilised more efficiently. For these practical reasons, 2-year studies are usually preferred. The pros and cons of assay sensitivity are much less clear cut. The longer that animals are allowed to live, the more likely they are to develop tumours and this is the main argument in favour of lifespan studies. However, losses due to cannibalism and autolysis may increase, as will the incidence of spontaneous background pathology. These confounding factors may negate the advantages of prolonging the study duration. This question of assay sensitivity cannot be answered in general terms, but can only be defined for one strain in one laboratory depending on the patterns of survival and spontaneous lesions that are expected under specified laboratory conditions. Thus, a lifespan (20–25% survival) study using the strain in Figure 4.18 would have a duration of approximately 2–5 years. Other strains may not reach the 25% survival point until after 3 years, significantly prolonging the duration and cost of a lifespan study.

Major causes

The pattern of causation of morbidity and mortality is equally as important as the rate. As discussed in Chapter 5, lethality or otherwise of tumours is important for tumour data analysis, but the pattern of all causes of morbidity and mortality is important because this pattern can be altered by treatment. In some cases, the pattern can be altered without any obvious change in survival rate. In other instances, the survival rate may be shortened or prolonged. The overall pattern of neoplastic and non-neoplastic causes of morbidity and mortality associated with the survival curve in Figure 4.18 is presented in Table 4.6.

Table 4.6.   Incidence (%) of non-neoplastic and neoplastic causes of morbidity and mortality in Sprague-Dawley rats at different study intervals (in weeks).

Cause	Male				Female			
	<52	52–78	79–104	>104	<52	52–78	79–104	>104
Non-neoplasia	82	32	37	36	39	7	6	7
Neoplasia	18	68	63	64	61	93	94	93

One feature of this summary table is that the general pattern of causation of morbidity and mortality in this strain does not change once the animals enter the second year of the study. Thus, at each time period studied after week 52 approximately one-third of the males will be necropsied because of non-neoplastic causes of illness and two-thirds because of neoplasms. Similarly, over 90% of females will be sent to necropsy because of neoplasia. This pattern is the reverse of that seen in man in which non-neoplastic lesions such as cardiovascular disease are the predominant causes of death.

The next patterns of interest are those within these two major causal groups. Lethal conditions can be split into two main types on the basis of frequency, namely common and uncommon conditions. If Table 4.6 is expanded slightly, the main subpatterns are as shown in Table 4.7. The subpatterns in females are simple. Approximately 80% of unscheduled necropsies are caused by two tumour types, pituitary and mammary, and this pattern is constant throughout the ageing period. Other lethal tumours considered on an individual organ basis account for less than 5% of morbidity and mortality, and a similar case holds for various types of non-neoplastic lesions. Pituitary tumours cause illness and death because of their critical position at the base of the brain, and relatively small tumours may be fatal. Mammary tumours are not critically located. These subcutaneous tumours may exceed 100 g without causing any apparent ill health unless they ulcerate or impede the animal's movement.

Table 4.7. Incidence (%) of morbidity and mortality in Sprague-Dawley rats due to the main groups of non-neoplastic and neoplastic causes. Results are given at different study intervals (in weeks).

Cause	Male			Female		
	52–78	79–104	>104	52–78	79–104	>104
Non-neoplasia						
Degenerations	8	8	12	2	1	0
Inflammations	8	8	8	2	2	2
Other conditions	2	2	8	1	1	5
Uncertain/multifactorial	14	19	8	2	2	0
Neoplasia						
Pituitary	40	30	21	45	41	45
Subcutis	19	13	16	1	2	2
Mammary	0	0	0	33	43	32
Other tumours	9	20	27	14	8	14

The causes of morbidity and mortality in males are more diverse. Two main tumour types, pituitary tumours and fibrous tumours of the subcutis, account for many losses, but the pattern is not as dominant as in females and several other tumour types occur. The incidence of these other lethal tumours tends to increase with time, but rarely exceeds 5% if they are considered on an individual tissue basis. Thus, the pattern of neoplastic losses in males has a certain constancy to it. Two tumours predominate and are accompanied with time by a slowly increasing range of low frequency tumour types such as bone tumours, liver tumours and various endocrine tumours.

About one-third of unscheduled necropsies in males are not associated with any large, ulcerated or critically situated neoplasms, and morbidity and mortality in these cases has to be attributed to non-neoplastic causes. In many cases, there may be no major morphological lesion to account for illness, or there may be two or more conditions of equivalent biological impact and the cause has to be stated as uncertain or multifactorial. In other cases, there may be major degenerative lesions in the kidney, nervous system or heart or inflammation in the skin, appendages or genitourinary tract and these together with other obvious lesions can be attributed unequivocally as the cause of the animal's demise. The pattern of these non-neoplastic causes of demise has a reasonable constancy with time, except that the uncertainty tends to decrease as the major degenerations associated with old age become more prominent. In some strains, particularly those fed high-protein diets *ad libitum*, kidney disease can be the major cause of morbidity and mortality in males.

Analysis of the incidence and causes of morbidity and mortality is not a common practice in long-term studies, but has much to commend it in assessing the biological significance of lesions. Changes in mortality rate or in the major patterns of causation are easily detected and are more likely to be relevant in risk assessment than any minor increases in the incidence of microscopic or small tumours found in groups of animals dying from other causes. The survival pattern in this particular strain of rat also suggests that assay sensitivity is unlikely to be increased by extending a study beyond 2 years. 2 years is approximately the 50% survival point and the patterns of causation after this point are relatively constant. These patterns are dominated by three or four major entities, and the sudden appearance of a biologically and statistically significant increase in other lesions in the remaining rats could be difficult to detect. Similar considerations apply to many other strains of rat. The majority of morbidity and mortality is usually dominated by a small number of non-neoplastic and neoplastic conditions throughout the ageing period.

Non-neoplastic lesions

An incidence summary table similar to that presented for young animals would fill several pages, and consideration of non-neoplastic pathology in the ageing rat is necessarily restricted to the more common and biologically significant lesions. The common lesions can be grouped into degenerative, inflammatory and proliferative lesions, the latter overlapping to some extent with neoplasms (Table 4.8). The paucity of entries in Table 4.8, which was derived from one containing over 200 diagnoses, illustrates that patterns of pathology in this and many other strains are dominated by a relatively small group of conditions. Most other lesions reported in ageing control rats are of low incidence and of minor biological significance. These are not discussed. Biological impact of a lesion is equally as important as frequency and the common lesions in Table 4.8 can be divided into two main groups on this basis. For example, degenerations of the kidney and nervous system can be lethal, whereas those in the liver and reproductive organs are usually incidental findings at necropsy. The main emphasis in this section will be on the clinically significant lesions and on lesions that cause problems in data analysis.

Non-neoplastic proliferations are a particular problem in analysis. The main use of long-term studies in rats is as a model bioassay for carcinogenicity. Non-neoplastic proliferations are seldom of clinical significance, but are extremely important because of the diagnostic difficulties they create in differentiation from preneoplastic lesions and from neoplasms. For example, spontaneous liver tumours are rare, but the liver is a common target organ of carcinogens and therefore spontaneous proliferations are important because they mask or mimic preneoplastic changes. In contrast, endocrine proliferations and tumours are common in rats, and the choice of criteria to differentiate non-neoplastic and neoplastic proliferations can profoundly alter the reported incidence of endocrine tumours in various laboratories.

Table 4.8.   Common non-neoplastic lesions in ageing Sprague-Dawley rats.

DEGENERATION	
Kidney	glomerulonephropathy
Nerve	radiculoneuropathy
Testis	atrophy
Ovary	atrophy/cyst
Liver	steatosis
	microcystic degeneration
	telangiectasis
INFLAMMATION	
Foot	pododermatitis/arthritis
Tail	dermatitis/folliculitis
Pancreas	pancreatitis
PROLIFERATION	
Liver	biliary proliferation
	altered cell foci/nodules
Adrenal	altered cell foci/nodules
Mammary	hyperplasia

Glomerulonephropathy

Of the degenerations, glomerulonephropathy is probably the number one non-neoplastic condition in the ageing rat in that it accounts for a significant proportion of morbidity and mortality. The severity of renal disease can be profoundly influenced by factors such as genotype and diet, and its presence hinders evaluation of chronic nephrotoxicity. Glomerulonephropathy has numerous synonyms, including nephropathy, nephrosis and glomerulonephrosis; and theories regarding its pathogenesis are equally numerous. The incidence and severity of disease are greater in males than in females. In advanced cases, the kidneys are enlarged, tan and irregular at necropsy and the cut surface in severe cases may be grossly cystic. Histologically, both glomerular and tubular changes are present, but the latter are dominant. Some tubules are shrunken with thickened basement membranes accompanied by variable degrees of interstitial fibrosis. Other tubules contain hyaline casts or form large cysts filled with proteinaceous material. Glomerular changes are relatively inconspicuous and are characterised mainly by varying degrees of sclerosis and cystic dilation of Bowman's space. Such severe cases are unusual in 2-year-old rats, and in most instances 50% or more of the kidney may appear reasonably normal.

The kidneys play a major role in fluid and electrolyte homeostasis and are used in the excretion of waste products. However, there is considerable reserve capacity and a rat may survive for a long time, even with severely distorted kidneys, before

dying of renal failure. Because the kidneys play a central role in fluid and electrolyte balance, advanced cases may lead to secondary patterns of pathology (syndromes) in other organs. The two main syndromes affect the cardiovascular system
and calcium/ phosphorus homeostasis (Figure 4.19).

The kidney receives 25% of the cardiac output and is intimately concerned
with blood pressure regulation through the renin–angiotensin system. It is not
surprising, therefore, that severe renal disease sometimes results in secondary cardiovascular disease. This may be expressed morphologically in the heart and
arteries. The most common finding is increased myocardial fibrosis especially
in the left ventricle. The more advanced cases may show left atrial thrombosis
or arteritis. Arteritis may be seen in one or more vessels, including renal vessels,
but is most commonly recorded in the pancreatic, mesenteric and testicular arteries.
Florid cases in mesenteric vessels can be seen at necropsy as blue tortuous or
nodular vessels in the mesentery around the duodenum and pancreas.
Histologically the affected vessels show varying degrees of thrombosis, aneurysmal
dilatation, fibrinoid necrosis and leucocyte infiltration.

The mineralisation syndrome is related to the kidney's role in calcium and
phosphorus homeostasis via control of tubular resorption, and also via synthesis
of the 1,25 dihydroxy-derivative of vitamin D_3. The pathogenesis of the syndrome is incompletely understood, but renal impairment results in hyper-
phosphataemia and acidosis. Calcium : phosphorus imbalance stimulates
parathyroid hyperplasia and there is increased bone resorption to correct the
hypocalcaemia. Severe cases can be defined at necropsy. The parathyroids are
grossly enlarged, the bones are thin and brittle and the aorta is dilated and rigid
due to mineral deposited in the media. This mineralisation affects many tissues
histologically and is known as metastatic mineralisation in contrast to the focal
dystrophic mineralisation (nephrocalcinosis) that is a common finding in the
young rat.

Glomerulonephropathy and its associated syndromes illustrate an important
point in database review. The incidence of lesions in toxicity studies is usually
summarised on an organ-by-organ basis, either alphabetically or by organ systems,
and biologically related lesions may appear in totally different places. The reviewing toxicologist or statistician must be aware of the common syndromes and should
not blindly consider every single entry on the summary table as an independent
entity. Equally important in such reviews is to acknowledge that the strength of
causal associations between lesions is variable. Thus, not every severe case of renal
disease results in arteritis nor is every case of arteritis caused by renal disease.

Radiculoneuropathy

The second major degenerative lesion in the ageing rat is radiculoneuropathy,
and this is another example of a small group of related lesions that may appear
in different parts of incidence summary tables. This disease may appear clinically
as minor ataxia or as hind limb paralysis with urinary incontinence in severe cases.
The lesion, like glomerulonephropathy, is predominant in males. Histologically,

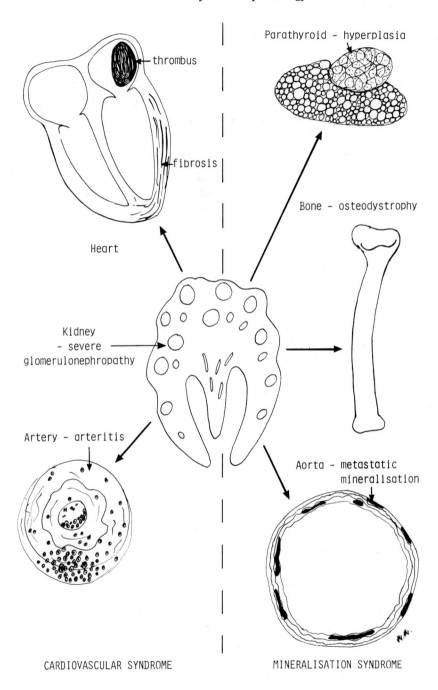

Figure 4.19. Secondary effects of severe glomerulonephropathy.

degeneration is seen in the posterior spinal cord (myelopathy), posterior nerve roots (radiculoneuropathy) and sciatic nerve (peripheral neuropathy) and results in secondary changes in the hind-limb muscles (atrophy). Paralysis and urinary incontinence may predispose to infection of the urogenital tract, resulting in inflammation of the prostate (prostatitis), bladder (cystitis) and kidney (pyelonephritis). These forms of -itis can be severe and fatal in contrast with the minor lesions in young animals, and illustrate the importance of qualifying terms in diagnoses.

Myelin, a lipid-rich material, is a major component of the nervous system and loss and removal of lipid accounts for most of the range of histological appearances of this degenerative disease. Swelling of myelin may produce vacuoles, degeneration produces myelin bodies (ovoids), digestion of lipid can be seen as foamy macrophages or in severe cases as cholesterol deposits (clefts) and astrocytic, Schwann cell or fibrocytic proliferation fills the space formerly occupied by the myelin (Figure 4.20).

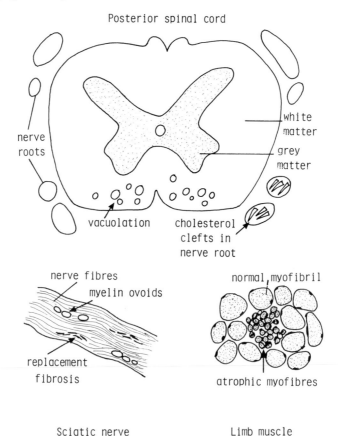

Figure 4.20. Radiculoneuropathy syndrome in old male rats.

Radiculoneuropathy is very common in ageing males, but usually asymptomatic. In contrast, there is a low-frequency degeneration of the anterior CNS which may produce obvious neurological symptoms and the animal has to be removed from the study. This condition termed encephalopathy, or more descriptively spongiform encephalopathy consists of a multifocal vacuolation of grey and white matter, most notable histologically in the cerebral cortex as a pale moth-eaten appearance. Minor cases can be easily masked by artefacts, but the brain of old rats showing acute neurological symptoms in the absence of pituitary or brain tumours should be examined carefully for this condition.

Testicular atrophy

Atrophy may appear as a primary condition in ageing rats, but is also secondary to large pituitary tumours and to testicular arteritis. This is an example of a condition which may appear as a single entry on an incidence summary table, but the incidence may be due to a variety of causes. Toxicologists and statisticians should be aware of the conditions where pooling data due to different causes is commonly done. Atrophy of seminiferous tubules ranges from focal unilateral to diffuse bilateral, and severe cases appear grossly as small, blue or brown, sometimes flaccid and watery gonads. Histologically the tubules are shrunken and the seminiferous epithelium is lost leaving only Sertoli cells (Figure 4.21). Interstitial oedema is also frequent, and Leydig cell hyperplasia may occur.

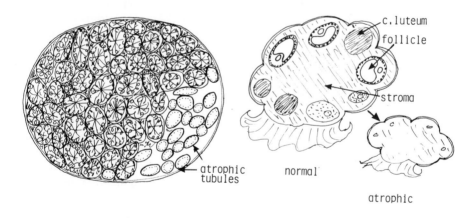

Focal testicular atrophy   Ovarian atrophy

Figure 4.21. Gonadal atrophy in ageing rats. C. =Corpus luteum.

Ovarian atrophy/cyst

This is usually bilateral and characterised by a decrease in number and size of follicles and corpora lutea, and an increase in the relative amount of stroma and interstitial tissue. The appearance of this remaining stroma is highly variable and may include nests of yellow pigmented cells, Sertoli-like tubules and tumour-like proliferations of spindle cells. Ovarian cysts are another common finding in ageing females. In contrast to those in the mouse, they are relatively small and appear as clear or yellow fluid-filled cysts about 10 mm in diameter. Histologically, they are usually simple unilocular cavities lined by flattened epithelium and appear to have little or no endocrine activity.

Hepatic steatosis

Steatosis in the liver is a very general term unless qualified further and includes both focal and diffuse change, the latter being either centrilobular or periportal. The appearance of fat droplets is equally variable and may be either macrocytic or microcytic. The pathogenesis of steatosis may be equally diverse and include dysfunction in the hepatocyte or imbalance in general lipid homeostasis. The latter is probably more common in ageing rats either because of obesity due to *ad libitum* feeding or due to lipid mobilisation in animals ill because of pituitary tumours or other debilitating lesions. In these cases, diffuse periportal steatosis is common. Like testicular atrophy, toxicologists should be aware that the incidence of steatosis due to different causes may be pooled for the presentation in summary tables.

Microcystic degeneration

This occurs in the liver and is also known as spongiosa hepatica. It may be visible at necropsy, but is usually a histological finding characterised by groups of thin-walled cysts, containing pale-pink proteinaceous material and occasionally a few erythrocytes (Figure 4.22). The microcysts are thought to be derived from the fat-storing (Ito) cell in the liver. They are found mainly in males.

Telangiectasis

This is another common liver lesion. It is a vascular lesion, but is probably secondary to or associated with atrophy of hepatic cords. It is most obvious at necropsy as depressed red foci on the surface of the liver and is particularly conspicuous when the liver is slightly yellow due to steatosis. Histologically, these foci are groups of dilated sinusoids usually located below the liver capsule (Figure 4.22). Telangiectasis is also very common in the adrenal cortex.

Pododermatitis/arthritis

Inflammations of major biological impact are uncommon in ageing rats unless they suffer from enzootic diseases such as mycoplasmosis. Prostatitis and other urogenital tract lesions are occasionally seen in animals with hind limb paralysis, but apart from these, lesions of the hind feet are the only common inflammations likely to make a significant impact on the health of the rat. Foot lesions are basically husbandry-related inflammations and are comprised of two main entities, pododermatitis and arthritis (Figure 4.23). Rats are commonly housed

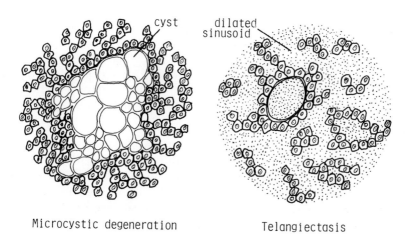

Microcystic degeneration   Telangiectasis

Figure 4.22. Degenerative lesions in ageing rat liver.

on grid or mesh floors and males may reach 1 kg in weight on *ad libitum* feeding. It is not surprising, therefore, that this combination of high body weight and mesh floors occasionally results in lesions of the feet, particularly in the heavier males. Up to 5% of ageing males may be removed from a study because of these two foot lesions.

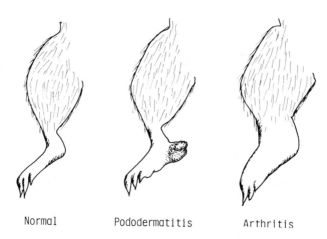

Normal   Pododermatitis   Arthritis

Figure 4.23. Gross appearance of hind-foot lesions in ageing male rats.

Pododermatitis is a local inflammation of the skin of the foot. It begins initially as a wart-like growth or callus on the foot pad due to continued pressure, and compensatory proliferation of the skin. However, infection, ulceration and bleeding may subsequently occur. Histologically, the lesion consists of inflamed granulation tissue variably covered by a hyperplastic squamous epithelium.

Arthritis is inflammation of the joint and surrounding tissues. Severe cases appear clinically as grossly swollen, firm, blue feet and hocks and may significantly impair the animal's mobility. The initial lesion is a periarthritis or tenosynovitis resulting in marked periarticular oedema with fibrosis and mononuclear leucocyte infiltration. The metatarsal joint ultimately becomes affected and in some cases the persistent chronic inflammation may incite a dramatic reactive bony proliferation which completely obscures the original skeletal architecture.

Dermatitis/folliculitis

Other inflammatory lesions of the skin and appendages also occur, but these are generally minor. The most common is inflammation of the hair follicle (folliculitis) in the tail. Nodules or pustules are frequent along the tail and are primarily a logistic problem related to good laboratory practice (GLP) rather than a clinical problem. Theoretically a tail nodule could be a tumour, and occasionally this is case, but the vast majority are various stages of suppurative folliculitis. Many long-term study protocols state that all gross lesions will be examined histologically and a histopathologist will rapidly become an expert on rat tails (and ears or feet) if this requirement is adhered to strictly. These appendigeal lesions could reasonably be treated in the same way as erect fur or fur loss in the skin, or as roundworms and tapeworms in the intestine. The clinical and necropsy data can be regarded as a definitive diagnosis in the vast majority of cases without the need to resort to histopathology.

Two other lesions of the integument pose similar problems. These are small nodules in the subcutis of the preputial region or on the back of males. These may be faithfully recorded week after week during the in-life phase of the study as palpable masses which grow slowly if at all, and some may regress. These two entities are preputial abscesses and squamous (epidermoid inclusion) cysts respectively. Repeated palpation may aggravate and rupture the lesions and necessitate removal of the animal from the study.

Pancreatitis

The last minor inflammatory lesion affects the pancreas. The histological appearance of this lesion is quite characteristic, but its status as a degenerative lesion (atrophy, microductular change) or post-inflammatory lesion (adenitis, pancreatitis) is ill-defined. There is focal loss of acinar epithelial cells producing a ductular structure often accompanied by a mild interstitial inflammatory response. The lesion may be multifocal, but most of the exocrine pancreas is normal.

Biliary proliferation

Focal proliferations of bile ducts are common in liver. They are generally minor histological observations. Biliary proliferation (bile duct hyperplasia) consists of clusters or chains of bile duct-like formations lined by cuboidal or flattened epithelium (Figure 4.24). The proliferations are generally in the vicinity of the portal triad and may show varying degrees of basement membrane thickening or fibrosis. These structures do not progress to neoplasia, but the more basophilic cellular lesions could possibly mimic early phase oval cell (ductular) hyperplasia which is a response sometimes observed in the liver of rats fed carcinogens.

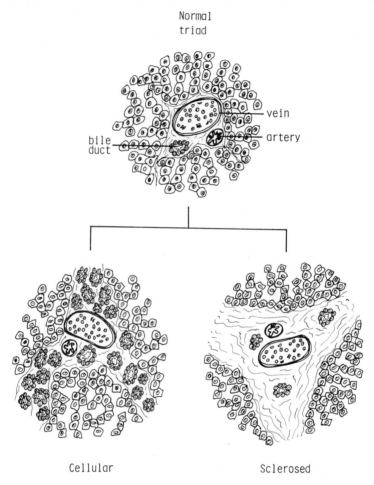

Figure 4.24. Biliary proliferation in rat liver.

Altered liver cell foci

These are a more controversial entity than biliary proliferation as a precursor of neoplasia. The focal proliferations consist of groups of hepatocytes which stand out from the normal liver parenchyma because of their arrangement, size or tinctorial properties. They also have biochemical and functional properties such as inability to store iron and increased γ-glutamyl-transpeptidase activity which differentiate them from normal hepatocytes. However, in routine HE paraffin sections they are usually classified into vacuolated (clear), acidophilic, basophilic or mixed cell foci (Figure 4.25).

Vacuolated cell foci are characterised by 'empty' cytoplasm representing the space occupied by glycogen or occasionally fat. The cells are usually larger than the surrounding hepatocytes. An increased amount of acidophilic cytoplasm is the characteristic feature of acidophilic foci, and the hepatocytes may also have an enlarged nucleus with a prominent nucleolus. In contrast, the hepatocytes forming basophilic foci are smaller than normal and the cytoplasm contains prominent clumps of basophilic granules. Mixed foci as the name suggests contain hepatocytes of two or more of the previous types. Foci exceeding the size of a hepatic lobule are sometimes called areas of cellular alteration, and ones larger still that compress the surrounding parenchyma may be referred to as nodules. Basophilic foci are the most common and are encountered mainly in ageing females. Overall, these altered cell foci and areas are uncommon in this strain of rat and do not significantly mask the interpretation of hepatocarcinogenic effects.

Altered adrenal cell foci

In contrast to the liver, altered cell foci areas and nodules are very common in the adrenal cortex, particularly in females. As in the liver, the lesions can be

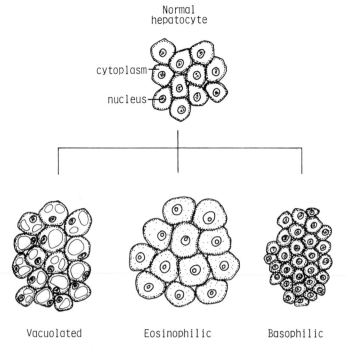

Figure 4.25. Altered cell foci in rat liver.

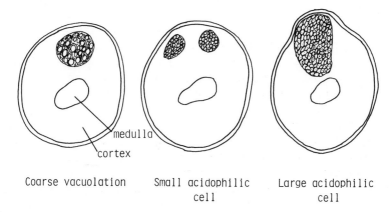

medulla

cortex

Coarse vacuolation   Small acidophilic   Large acidophilic
                             cell   cell

Figure 4.26. Altered cell foci in rat adrenal cortex.

classified on the basis of staining characteristics into vacuolated, acidophilic, basophilic etc., although there are subclasses of each type (Figure 4.26).

Finely vacuolated foci are found in both sexes and usually affect the zona glomerulosa and outer zona fasciculata. Coarsely vacuolated foci are most common in males and usually lie in the central zona fasciculata. The small acidophilic cell focus (sometimes called hyperplastic focus) is often multiple and in the outer zona fasciculata. The lesion of most concern is the large acidophilic cell focus. These proliferations are common in ageing females and may grow to grossly visible nodules of debatable diagnostic classification. They provide a useful example of the diagnostic uncertainty that exists in toxicological pathology.

The two main criteria used in the classification of proliferations as tumours are morphology and the probability of progression. Morphological criteria include atypical cytology and organisation. Nuclear : cytoplasmic ratio, tinctorial properties, anaplasia and mitotic rate are the main cytological characteristics that distinguish neoplastic cells from normal cells. Organisational atypia includes abnormal growth patterns, compression or invasion, and abnormal relationships between proliferating cells and blood vessels or other mesenchymal elements. These patterns serve to differentiate neoplasms from non-neoplastic proliferations.

Probability criteria are mathematical assessments of the degree of association between small lesions of debatable classification and large clear-cut neoplasms. Crudely stated, if large, lethal masses are common in an organ then common microscopic lesions are probably microscopic tumours or at least precursor lesions with a high probability of neoplastic transformation. On the other hand, if microscopic foci are common and gross tumours are rare in old animals, there is a low probability of any biologically significant degree of progressive growth suggestive of neoplastic transformation. Pathologists use all of these criteria in assessing proliferations, but with different degrees of emphasis. This results in highly variable incidence data for certain types of proliferation. The reviewing toxicologist must become familiar with the main problem areas in which one man's hyperplasia is another man's neoplasia and evaluate the data in the full knowledge of this diagnostic uncertainty.

If the above criteria are applied to the large acidophil proliferations in the adrenal cortex, then on a morphological basis large compressing nodules of cytologically distinct cells, sometimes with frequent mitoses, are common in the female adrenal. On this basis, there could be a 40% or more incidence of cortical tumours in some rat strains. Alternatively, the probable fate of many of these proliferations is to undergo vacuolar degeneration resulting in a large blood-filled cyst which may thrombose (Figure 4.27). Further evidence against a neoplastic diagnosis is that large undoubted cortical neoplasms are often composed of small acidophilic cells cytologically distinct from the hypertrophied acidophilic cell of the commonly occurring nodules. Thus, if diagnosis is based on this cytological discontinuity and the high incidence of degeneration, these nodules would be regarded as hyperplastic rather than neoplastic.

The proliferation of hyperbasophilic phaeochromocytes in the adrenal medulla is an example of classification in the other direction. In this case, these is a reasonable continuity in both cytology and incidence to suggest progression from small basophilic foci to large metastasing proliferations in rats nearing the end of their lifespan (Figure 4.28). Similar continuities are seen in the anterior

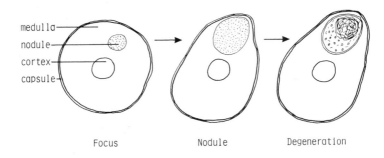

Figure 4.27. Probable progression of many acidophilic nodules in rat adrenal cortex.

pituitary and in the C-cell population of the thyroid. In all these cases, foci may be considered adenomas even though they are small, non- compressing and with infrequent mitoses. There is no easy answer to these diagnostic problems, but they are often at the centre of controversial conclusions from carcinogenicity studies. It cannot be stressed too frequently that toxicologists and statisticians should appreciate the level of uncertainty that surrounds the classification of microscopic proliferations as hyperplasias or as neoplasias and evaluate the data accordingly.

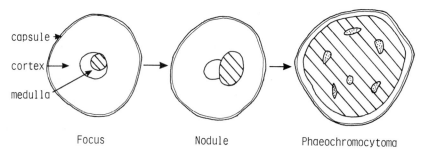

Figure 4.28. Probable progression of basophilic foci in the rat adrenal medulla.

Neoplasia

The incidence and types of neoplasia are usually the patterns of pathology of most concern in long-term studies. The pattern of common tumours in this particular strain at 2 years of age is presented in Table 4.9. The pattern is dominated by subcutaneous connective tissue tumours, mammary proliferations and by endocrine tumours. Other tumour types occur at incidence rates of less than 10% and in most cases rarely exceed 3%.

Table 4.9. Percentage 2-year-old rats bearing specific tumour types.

Tissue	Tumour	Male	Female
Skin subcutis	Connective tissue tumour	26	8
	Mammary tumour	1	55
Endocrine system	Pituitary tumour	62	76
	Thyroid C-cell tumour	21	19
	Adrenal phaeochromocytoma	24	3

Subcutaneous tumours

Large subcutaneous masses are a common finding in ageing rats and may exceed 100 g in weight. In males, a variety of connective-tissue tumours occurs, but they are usually fatty or fibrous, the latter predominating. Fatty tumours (lipomas) are seen at necropsy as large, smooth, soft, glistening masses and are most easily defined in debilitated animals when the normal subcutaneous adipose tissue is depleted. In obese males, the distinction between small lipomas and large fat depots is not clear cut. Histologically, the lipoma consists of mature lipocytes sometimes with small bands of fibrosis.

Large, well-differentiated fibromas are the predominant subcutaneous connective tissue in males. Large tumours may impede movement or become ulcerated and the animal has to be removed from the study. They appear grossly as well circumscribed, firm, multinodular masses with a variable appearance on cut surface ranging from uniform white to a mosaic of white, cream pink and red areas. The histological appearance may vary widely within different areas of the same tumour. Fibroblasts are elongated cells producing collagen and ground substance and the histological appearance of tumours depends on the arrangement of the cells and the relative proportion of cells to cell product. Most tumours contain abundant collagen, but in some areas ground substance may predominate producing a myxomatous appearance (Figure 4.29). The more cellular areas may suggest malignant transformation, but the fate of these cells appears to be differentiation rather than progression to fibrosarcoma since cellular areas are common and metastases from these large subcutaneous masses are virtually non-existent. Fibrosarcomas do occur, but are not common. Their characteristic histological feature is basophilia due to uniform hypercellularity in contrast to the largely eosinophilic fibroma. Mitotic figures are frequent and some tumours contain bizarre giant cells and multinucleate cells.

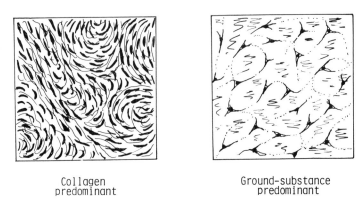

Collagen
predominant   Ground-substance
                         predominant

Figure 4.29. Variation in rat subcutaneous fibromas.

Another frequently encountered, but generally small mass is the dermal fibroma. This is a distinct entity composed of an irregular mass of coarse collagen fibres similar to those of the normal dermis. Larger nodules extend into the subcutis. Both small and large nodules may contain sufficient adipose tissue to justify the combined diagnosis fibrolipoma (Figure 4.30). The relationship of

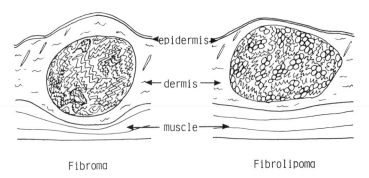

Fibroma   Fibrolipoma

Figure 4.30. Dermal tumours in the male rat.

this tumour to the large subcutaneous fibroma is uncertain, but it is probably a separate entity rather than a precursor lesion.

Mammary tumours

Subcutaneous masses are more common in females than in males. They are frequently multiple and usually mammary in origin. The gross and histological appearance of these tumours is highly variable, but the majority are variants of a single entity, mammary fibroadenoma. The rat has six pairs of mammary glands consisting of milk-secreting epithelium and supporting or contractile stroma. Both epithelial and stromal elements proliferate, hence the diagnosis fibroadenoma. The degree of proliferation often varies in different parts of the same tumour, resulting in areas that are predominantly fibrous, predominantly epithelial or mixed fibroepithelial. Diagnostic terms such as adenofibroma or fibroadenoma may be used to reflect the relative proportions of each component, but this division is probably unnecessary. Purely fibrous tumours may be impossible to distinguish from subcutaneous fibromas on one single section, but glandular formations may be found if multiple samples of the mass are examined. For statistical classification it is reasonable to consider fibrous tumours in females as a variant of mammary fibroadenoma (Figure 4.31).

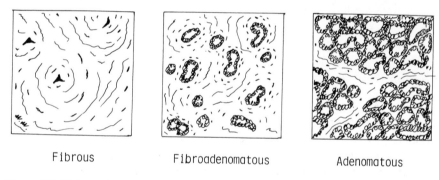

| Fibrous | Fibroadenomatous | Adenomatous |

Figure 4.31. Variation in rat mammary fibroadenoma.

Pituitary tumours

Subcutaneous masses are the tumours most frequently seen as 'palpable masses' in the in-life phase of long-term studies, but endocrine tumours are just as frequent in the final pathology phase. This group is dominated by the pituitary adenoma both in incidence and biological significance. Pituitary tumours are frequently visible at necropsy and are a common cause of morbidity and mortality. Thyroid C-cell tumours and adrenal phaeochromocytomas are less common and frequently microscopic entities.

The anterior pituitary secretes several hormones and pituicytes fall into three main groups, acidophilic, basophilic and chromophobe depending on the tinctorial properties of the cytoplasm. In the past, attempts were made to use tinctorial classifications in the diagnosis of pituitary tumours, but this has largely been abandoned in favour of the non-specific diagnosis 'pituitary adenoma' or 'pituitary tumour'. More sophisticated investigational techniques such as ultrastructure, immunocytochemistry and hormone assay suggest that the majority of tumours secrete prolactin and the term prolactinoma is sometimes used. However, in routine HE sections it is impossible to delineate functional properties and inappropriate to use specific terms without any evidence for the functional status of the tumour.

Pituitary tumours range in size from microscopic to macroscopic (Figure 4.32) and this raises once again the question of hyperplasia versus neoplasia. Since large lethal tumours 10mm or more in diameter are common in this strain, the equally common microscopic lesions of similar cytology, but just smaller in terms of size can reasonably be considered in the spectrum of adenomas. The microscopic appearance varies. In females, the cells are generally small to medium in size with relatively little cytoplasm (chromophobes). Dilated vascular channels are frequent and haemosiderin pigment is sometimes found. In males the cytology is much more diverse and bizarre pale eosinophilic cells are often seen. Microscopic tumours may be multicentric, and the larger tumours are nodular masses compressing the brain, often causing hydrocephalus. Most tumours are considered benign even though the cytology may be bizarre. Invasion of the meninges and along vascular channels into the brain is occasionally seen, but metastases are extremely rare.

The large tumours are space occupying and often functional and frequently result in other histological lesions. In females, acinar hyperplasia of the mammary gland and ovarian atrophy are commonly associated with pituitary neoplasms. Testicular atrophy may occur in males. Other components of the pituitary syndrome are splenic atrophy with haemosiderosis, squamous hyperplasia of the forestomach and steatosis in the liver. The clinical syndrome of a thin, neurologically abnormal rat with red tear stains around the eyes is almost pathognomonic of large pituitary tumours.

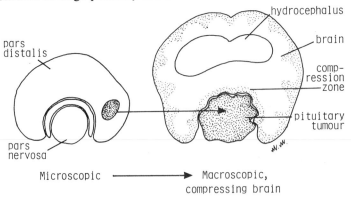

Figure 4.32. Pituitary adenoma in the rat.

C-cell tumours

The thyroid C-cell proliferations are slightly more of a diagnostic problem than those in the pituitary. A minor degree of diffuse proliferation is common and is usually termed hyperplasia. Focal proliferations range from single perifollicular aggregates to grossly visible masses. Terminology varies, but proliferations occupying large areas of the thyroid are common and the smaller foci could reasonably be considered part of the adenoma spectrum (Figure 4.33). However, other diagnoses used range from nodular hyperplasia to microscopic carcinoma depending on the diagnostic criteria applied by different pathologists. The data in Table 4.9 assume most proliferations to be C-cell adenomas. The cells usually form large pale acidophilic nests of round cells, compressing adjacent thyroid follicles. The larger tumours tend to incite fibrous encapsulation and occasionally show focal invasion of the capsule, surrounding tissues or metastasis to the cervical nodes. These large masses are designated carcinomas although the cytology and mitotic rate may not markedly differ from the smaller proliferations. Hence the tendency for some pathologists to refer to all proliferations as carcinoma.

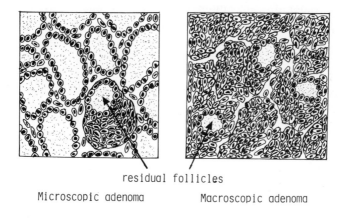

residual follicles

Microscopic adenoma Macroscopic adenoma

Figure 4.33. Thyroid C-cell tumour in the rat.

Phaeochromocytomas

These medullary proliferations were discussed earlier as part of the adrenal proliferations. They present the same diagnostic problems as thyroid and pituitary tumours, and the only point of comment is that in this strain they occur predominantly in males.

Other tumours

A diverse range of epithelial and mesenchymal tumours occurs in other tissues, and to the pathologist this creates fascinating diagnostic problems. The reviewing toxicologist, however, need only treat these as low-frequency tumour types. Since the prevalence of these tumours is usually below 3%, 10%, ie. five cases in a single sex group of 50 rats, is a useful cut-off point. Fewer than five cases is unlikely to be statistically significant (Chapter 5). The toxicologist has to rely on the subjective evaluation of the pathologist to interpret the biological significance of these low-frequency tumour types.

Summary

Pathology data bases in a long-term rat study can appear extremely complex, and in volume may account for the bulk of a toxicology report. Fortunately, the data are usually dominated by a small handful of entities and if these can be defined, the process of data review is much simplified. For example, this strain of Sprague-Dawley rat has a 50% survival time of approximately 2 years, and morbidity and mortality is due mainly to neoplasia, in particular to large sub-cutaneous masses or small, but critically located pituitary tumours. Overall, much of the pathology is associated with abnormalities in the endocrine system and endocrine-dependent tissues, plus a degree of degeneration in the kidney and nervous system. If the major patterns are known it is easy to classify treatment-related effects into those affecting common spontaneous lesions and those associated with unusual lesions. This is an important step in the early stages of data evaluation.

Finally, it is important to re-emphasise that variation between strains of rat or even between the same strain in different laboratories is remarkable although endocrine-related lesions or glomerulonephropathy usually dominate the picture. Variation also occurs between pathologists in their use of diagnostic criteria and toxicologists should be aware of the uncertain nature of incidence data, particularly regarding the common microscopic proliferations. Pathologists also vary in their approach to categorising and pooling data for incidence summary tables and this has an impact on statistical analyses. In some cases, a lesion may have several different causes and the total incidence due to all causes may be presented. Other lesions are linked as part of a generalised syndrome, but may appear as independent entries on a summary table.

The ageing mouse

The mouse is usually the second rodent species of choice for long-term studies. Longevity is usually slightly less than in rats. The incidence and severity of lesions increase with age and, as in the rat, the pattern varies from strain to strain. The CD-1 mouse maintained in one laboratory for 80 weeks or more on *ad libitum* feeding regimens will be the reference strain for this section.

Morbidity and mortality

The rate and causation of morbidity and mortality in the mouse are more complex than in the rat, but nevertheless, several major features can be identified.

Rate

The overall pattern of survival of the mouse is shown in Figure 4.34. Husbandry has such a major effect on the survival of males that two plots are required, single-housed and group-housed animals. The pattern in females is affected relatively little by housing density. Approximately 95% of single-housed mice are alive at the end of the first year of the study and then losses increase steadily to leave approximately 50% alive at the end of the second year. Under these conditions, males survive slightly better than females. However, in group-housed males, there is a greater attrition rate during the first year and as numbers subsequently decline during the second year, only 20–25% are alive at week 104.

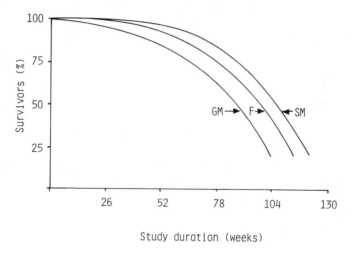

Study duration (weeks)

Figure 4.34. Survival curves for conventionally housed CD-1 mice 6–8 weeks old at study initiation. SM and GM = Single and group-housed males respectively; F = Females.

These survival patterns in males have a significant effect on protocol design and costs in long-term mouse studies. Conventional study durations are 80 weeks, 104 weeks and lifespan. A lifespan study in group-housed males would be about 104 weeks. In single-house studies over 50% of males would be alive at this point. Therefore, the study would have to be extended to about 130 weeks if a lifespan duration was designated in the protocol. Single housing is more costly than group housing and the extra cost of a further 6 months' housing is a significant proportion of the overall study cost.

Major causes

Fighting and urogenital tract lesions are the major cause of the increased morbidity and mortality in group-housed males, but this is only one factor in the overall pattern of non-neoplastic and neoplastic causes of morbidity and mortality. In contrast to the rat, non-neoplastic conditions have at least the same importance as neoplasia as causes of demise. Approximately equal numbers of the females die of neoplastic and non-neoplastic conditions throughout the ageing period (Table 4.10). In males, the pattern is more complex because of the effects of husbandry. When data from single- and group-housed animals are pooled there is a slight excess of morbidity and mortality due to non-neoplastic causes.

Table 4.10   Incidence (%) of non-neoplastic and neoplastic causes of morbidity and mortality in CD-1 mice at different study intervals (in weeks)

Cause	Male			Female		
	<52	52–80	>80	<52	52–80	>80
Non-neoplasia	79	65	60	50	50	54
Neoplasia	21	35	40	50	50	46

A wide range of specific causes of morbidity and mortality can be identified in a long-term mouse study. These conditions are described in more detail later, but like the rat the range tends to be dominated by a fairly small number of entities (Table 4.11). Approximately half of the females and slightly fewer males are removed from the study because of neoplasia. The predominant feature in females is neoplasia of the haemolymphoreticular tissues, particularly in the first 80 weeks

Table 4.11   Incidence (%) of morbidity and mortality in CD-1 mice due to the main groups of non-neoplastic and neoplastic causes at different study intervals (in weeks)

Cause	Male			Female		
	<52	52–80	>80	<52	52–80	>80
Non-neoplasia						
Skin-lesion	19	11	5	4	3	3
Urogenital tract lesion	31	24	21	—	—	—
Amyloidosis	0	12	11	0	16	15
Glomerulonephropathy	1	1	2	11	7	4
Haemorrhagic ovarian cyst	—	—	—	2	5	14
Other lesions	8	10	9	17	13	11
Uncertain/multifactorial	20	7	12	16	6	7
Neoplasia						
Haemolymphoreticular	13	16	9	39	30	18
Liver	1	9	15	0	1	1
Lung	0	5	8	2	2	4
Blood vessels	0	2	3	0	5	5
Uterus	—	—	—	2	4	9
Mammary	—	—	—	2	5	4
Other tumours	7	3	5	5	3	5

of the study. Beyond 80 weeks, other lethal tumours begin to increase, notably in the uterus. Haemolymphoreticular tumours also predominate in males, but-not to the same extent as in females and as the study progresses, there is a rising incidence of morbidity and mortality due to lung and liver neoplasms.

In group-housed males, a large proportion of the causes of non-neoplastic morbidity and mortality is due to lesions of the skin and urogenital tract. These are related mainly, but not exclusively to fighting. The skin lesions occur mainly on the head and neck, often as torn or bleeding ears or as ulcerative dermatitis extending around the neck. The latter may also be related to repeated handling by technicians, to scratching, or to abrasion between the animal and its cage and food hopper.

The genital area is another attack zone of aggressive males, but in this case skin lesions often lead to secondary changes in the urogenital tract and are conveniently encompassed in the overall term urogenital tract lesions. Such lesions include ulcerative dermatitis, preputial abscesses and lesions of the penis. These in themselves may be sufficiently severe to cause the animal to be removed from the study. In other cases minor lesions may lead to obstruction or to inflammation of the urogenital tract, and ascending pyelonephritis is a common sequel. Skin and urogential tract lesions are less frequent in the younger single-housed mice, and hence their better survival rate. However, urogenital tract lesions still cause a significant proportion of morbidity and mortality in males in studies over 80 weeks' duration. Amyloidosis is the other main cause of illness and death in males, largely because of the critical effects of amyloid deposited in renal glomeruli.

Amyloidosis is also a major non-neoplastic cause of demise in females, but in addition to renal failure due to amyloid, a significant proportion of females also develops renal failure as a result of glomerulonephropathy. The only other common lesion in females is haemorrhage into the large ovarian cysts that are frequent in females over 18 months of age. As in the rat, there are cases where no obvious lesions may be found to explain an animal's illness or several lesions may appear to contribute to an animal's demise. These tend to predominate in the early parts of a study, but overall the incidence of uncertain or multifactorial causes is only about 10% of all cases sent to necropsy.

Non-neoplastic lesions

A wide variety of non-neoplastic lesions are encountered in ageing mice, but only the more frequent and important groups are shown in Table 4.12. These common lesions can be divided into two main groups on the basis of biological significance to the health of the animals, and the emphasis in this section is on the clinically significant lesions.

Amyloidosis

The two major degenerations in CD-1 mice are amyloidosis and glomerulonephropathy, both of which may lead to renal failure or death. The grouping of these two conditions as degenerations is somewhat questionable as

Table 4.12. Common non-neoplastic lesions in ageing CD-1 mice.

DEGENERATION	
Connective tissue	amyloidosis
Kidney	glomerulonephropathy
	cortical cyst
Eye	retinal atrophy
Brain	mineralisation
Adrenal	pigment
Joint	arthrosis
Nerve	neuropathy
Testis	atrophy
Ovary	cyst
	atrophy
INFLAMMATION	
Skin	dermatitis
Urogenital	various lesions
PROLIFERATION	
Uterus	cystic hyperplasia
Adrenal	subcapsular hyperplasia
Stomach	adenomatous hyperplasia
Spleen	haemopoiesis
Lymphoid tissue	hyperplasia
Thymus	hyperplasia

proliferation could be arguably a prime factor in the disease. Amyloid, for example, is a fibrillar proteinaceous material deposited in the connective tissue around blood vessels. These protein deposits are presumably the result of excess protein synthesis and amyloid may therefore be considered the manifestation of a proliferative disease. Classically, amyloidosis is divided into primary and secondary types. In primary amyloidosis, the cause of the lesion is unknown, whereas secondary amyloidosis is frequently related to persistent chronic inflammation, which in mice is usually chronic dermatitis. This classical division is broadly consistent with the classification of amyloidosis on the basis of its major protein constituents. There are several different amyloid proteins, but primary amyloidosis is associated mainly with polypeptide chains derived from immunoglobulins, and secondary amyloid appears to b~ derived from the acute-phase reactants of plasma.

Amyloidosis in the CD-1 mouse is mainly a primary condition and is probably associated with disorders in the immune system. The disease primarily affects older mice and occurs in both sexes with a tendency to be more frequent as a cause of death in females than in males. Histologically, the proteins appear as amorphous pale acidophilic deposits. Many tissues may be affected, but it is usually associated with blood vessels of the large pore-type used in macromolecular transfer. Thus, sinusoids are common sites for deposits as are the lamina propria of the small intestine and the renal glomeruli. The latter site is most critical to the animal's well-being. Large deposits interfere with renal and cardiovascular function and death may be due to secondary degenerative renal changes (amyloid nephropathy) or to atrial thrombosis.

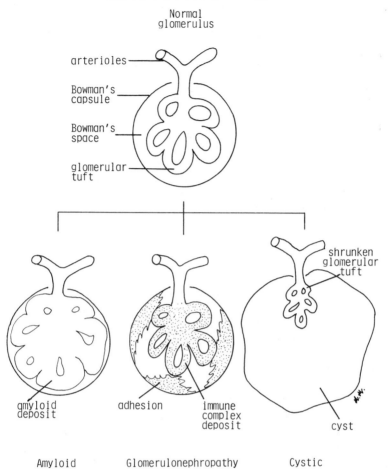

Figure 4.35. Glomerular conditions in mice.

Glomerulonephropathy

Also termed glomerulosclerosis or glomerulonephritis this is primarily a disease of females, and in contrast to amyloid is a significant condition in the young female accounting for about 10% of losses during the first year. Marked sub-cutaneous oedema in a young female is almost pathognomic of this lesion in its advanced form. Histologically, the glomeruli are obliterated by an intense acidophilic material rather than the pale acidophilic deposits characteristic of amyloid. The deposits may also be irregular and the glomeruli may appear distorted and shrunken, often with adhesions in contrast to the uniform enlarge-ment generally associated with amyloid. Secondary tubular lesions and car-diovascular complications such as oedema, arteritis and atrial thrombosis are common in advanced cases. This condition is very common in some strains of mice and appears to be associated with immune complex deposition. Thus, both of the main renal lesions in CD-1 mice appear to be immune-associated disorders.

Ocular degenerations

Retinal atrophy is the most common eye lesion, but lens cataracts and subepithelial mineralisation of the central cornea are also frequent (Figure 4.36). Retinal atrophy is primarily a histological lesion characterised by progressive loss of the rod and cone layer. It may occur in response to excessive artificial lighting or be secondary to lens cataracts. Cataracts are due mainly to swelling of the lens fibres and advanced cases are detectable clinically as opacities. Large areas of corneal mineralisation (dystrophy) may also be seen clinically, but the usual presentation is as a minor histological lesion.

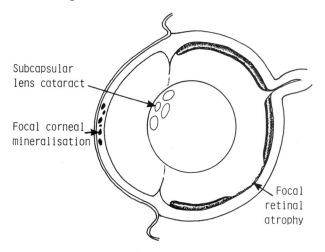

Figure 4.36. Eye lesions in ageing mice.

Arthrosis

Joint disease differs from the inflammatory distal extremity lesion encountered in the rat. In the mouse, it is a degenerative disease termed osteoarthrosis or simply arthrosis and affects mainly the larger weight-bearing joints such as the knee. It is primarily a disease of the ageing male and advanced cases may be detected clinically as bony nodules on the joint. Mobility is rarely impaired to an extent that requires the mouse to be removed from the study and the condition can be considered of relatively minor biological effect. However, it is a very common condition and the histological appearance may be very striking. Degeneration and erosion of articular cartilage are accompanied by bony proliferation at the joint margins resulting in the 'knobbly knees' of the advanced cases (Figure 4.37).

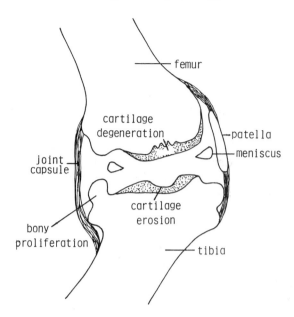

Figure 4.37. Arthrosis in the knee of an ageing male.

Other degenerations

A common minor renal degeneration in CD-1 mice is cystic dilation of Bowman's space. These cysts occur mainly in ageing males, are often multiple and the larger ones may be visible on the surface of the kidney at necropsy.

Mineralisation in the brain is a minor histological lesion located fairly specifically in blood vessels in the thalamus. The incidence depends largely on the plane of section routinely sampled in the laboratory. A more extensive pigment deposition occurs in the adrenal. Histologically, this is a brown pigment, resembling ceroid, deposited in the corticomedullary region. This occurs mainly in females and may appear as a wide band of brown pigment often referred to as 'brown degeneration'.

Peripheral nerve degeneration (neuropathy) is not nearly as common as in the rat, nor as severe, and it is rarely associated with clinical symptoms. Thus, in contrast to the rat it is a lesion of minor biological significance and is a further illustration of the importance of qualifying terms in diagnosis.

The remaining common degenerations affect the reproductive tract. Testicular atrophy is similar to that seen in the rat and is generally of little biological significance. Ovarian cysts are also of little significance in the younger female, but as the cysts enlarge with age they may reach 20 mm or more in diameter, and haemorrhage into the cyst may be fatal. Mice with renal glomerular lesions may be predisposed to ovarian cyst haemorrhage because of potential increases in blood pressure. Atrophy of the cycling ovarian elements is also common in ageing females, but, as in the rat, may be accompanied by pronounced proliferation of the stromal and interstitial tissues to produce a tumour-like condition.

Inflammations

The two major inflammatory conditions of the mouse — dermatitis and urogenital tract disease — were described under morbidity and mortality as they account for a significant proportion of male losses. Ulcerative dermatitis is a fairly consistent histological entity whether on the skin or on the appendages, but urogenital tract lesions may manifest themselves in a variety of ways. They may be predominantly inflammatory, or predominantly obstructive, or a combination of both. However, they can all be reasonably grouped into the same general category of lower urogenital tract disease.

Cystic endometrial hyperplasia

The range of common non-neoplastic proliferations encountered in the mouse is relatively small, and like the rat there is the same problem of differentiating between hyperplasias and neoplasias in some cases. One of the least controversial is cystic hyperplasia of the uterus. The endometrium of the mouse uterus is very sensitive to oestrogens and cystic hyperplasia is probably the sequel to persistent hormonal imbalance. A major, but probably not the only aetiological factor is the high incidence of ovarian cysts in ageing mice. Advanced cases may cause abdominal swelling and appear at necropsy as grossly enlarged firm convoluted uterine horns. Histologically, there is polypoid proliferation of the endometrium with large cystic glands and an oedematous endometrial stroma (Figure 4.38). Distorted and dilated vascular channels are a fairly common accompaniment and a fatal haemorrhage sometimes occurs.

Gastric adenomatous hyperplasia

The other major, but less frequent, mucosal proliferation of the ageing mouse is adenomatous hyperplasia of the glandular region of the stomach (Figure 4.38). As the name implies, the status of this lesion is uncertain. Many cases are microscopic lesions, but advanced forms appear at necropsy as a diffuse, sometimes polypoid thickening of the mucosa. Histologically, the epithelial proliferation often results in cystic structures which may extend downward into the submucosa or muscularis. Although this is suggestive of neoplasia, spread beyond the serosa is very rare and the status of this proliferation remains equivocal.

Adrenal subcapsular proliferations

The same equivocal status also applies to proliferations of the subcapsular cells in the adrenal. This is an extremely common and generally microscopic lesion that occurs mainly in the females of this strain. Two basic types of proliferation are found: focal and nodular. The focal proliferations are often multiple and bilateral and consist mainly of aggregates of small basophilic spindle cells (Type

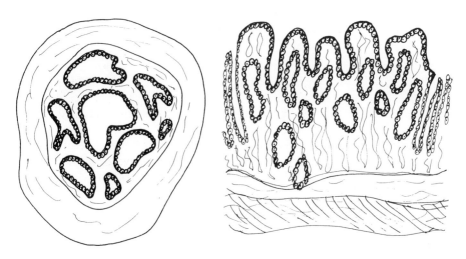

Cystic hyperplasia   Adenomatous hyperplasia
   of the uterus   of the stomach

Figure 4.38. Mucosal proliferations in the ageing mouse.

A) extending from the capsule into the cortex (Figure 4.39). The second form of proliferating subcapsular cell is the plump lipoidal cell (Type B). These are sometimes seen as small nests, but are more commonly encountered as the major component of nodules admixed with a small proportion of spindle cells. Nodules of lipoidal cells are usually solitary and may show extension over the surface of the adrenal. Such cases may be considered to be tumours, but there is no clear consensus on the true status of these nodular proliferations, particularly the smaller ones.

Haemolymphoreticular proliferations

The final group of non-neoplastic proliferations affects the haemolymphoreticular system and is of major importance in the pathology of the ageing mouse. This system is a complex structure anatomically, cytologically and functionally (Figure 4.40). As implied in the name it consists of three major and overlapping organisations: the haem-, lymph- and reticular-systems. The haem-system, or more appropriately the haemopoietic tissue, is located primarily in the bone marrow and in adult life is concerned mainly with production of two of the main cellular components of blood, erythrocytes and polymorphonuclear leucocytes. The precursor cells in the bone marrow are known as the erythroid and myeloid series respectively and the proportion of the two series in the marrow is usually in the range 1 : 2 to 2 : 1 (erythroid : myeloid ratio). In contrast to man and larger mammals, the bone marrow is very active throughout life and is frequently

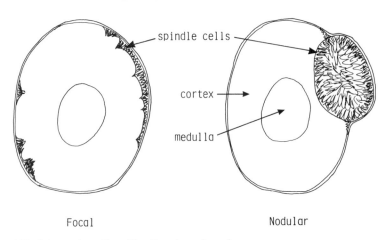

Figure 4.39. Subcapsular cell proliferations in ageing mice.

supported by production outside the marrow, a process termed extramedullary haemopoiesis. The red pulp of the spleen is the primary site of extramedullary haemopoiesis, and in the mouse the bone marrow and splenic red pulp can be considered the two main anatomical components of the haemopoietic system.

The lymph- component of haemolymphoreticular system is located mainly, but not exclusively outside the marrow and represented anatomically by the thymus, lymph nodes, splenic white pulp and epithelial-associated lymphoid nodules such as Peyer's patches in the small intestine. The main cytological components of the lymphoid system are lymphocytes, which are grouped into two main classes, B cells and T cells. There are complex functional interactions between these two cell types, but B cells are primarily associated with humoral immunity and T cells with cellular immune responses. These two functional classes have anatomical equivalents in the lymphoid tissues, for example, as the germinal centre and paracortical zones for B and T cells respectively.

The term 'reticular' is derived from the anatomical organisation known as the reticuloendothelial system and has the macrophage (histiocyte) as its main cellular component. Because the macrophage is a mononuclear leucocyte and its main functional role is phagocytosis, the modern tendency is to refer to this system as the mononuclear phagocyte system (MPS). In contrast to the haemopoietic and lymphopoietic tissues, the MPS is a diffuse organisation forming a small component of many organs. Within the concept of the haemolymphoreticular system, the main components are the sinusoidal phagocytic cells of the liver (Kupffer cells), spleen and lymph nodes, and the dendritic reticular cells of the lymphoid germinal centres.

All three components of the haemolymphoreticular system may proliferate, sometimes independently, and sometimes in various combinations. This complexity is further confounded by the variable cytology of any one particular cell line. For example, proliferating lymphoid cells may appear as small lymphocytes, plasma cells, immunoblasts and large undifferentiated blast cells or any combination of these types. In addition, autolysis rapidly obscures many of the cytological distinctions between different cell types. This complexity and variability, together with the inherent problem in any tissue of differentiating between hyperplasia and neoplasia makes the study of haemolymphoreticular proliferations very difficult even for the most experienced pathologist. Thus, a toxicologist or a statistician reviewing numerical incidence summary data should be acutely aware of the degree of uncertainty surrounding some of the data on the haemolymphoreticular system of the ageing mouse.

Perhaps the most clear-cut non-neoplastic haemolymphoreticular proliferation is increased haemopoiesis in the splenic red pulp. A small amount of haemopoiesis is normal in the spleen, but proliferation occurs rapidly in response to increased demand. The three main causes of increased demand are inflammation, haemorrhage and neoplasia. Inflammatory lesions are common in the skin and urogenital tract of males and are frequently accompanied by an enlarged spleen producing mainly myeloid cells. Myelopoiesis is also seen in females, but erythroid-dominant haemopoiesis is also frequent as part of the haemopoietic response to vascular

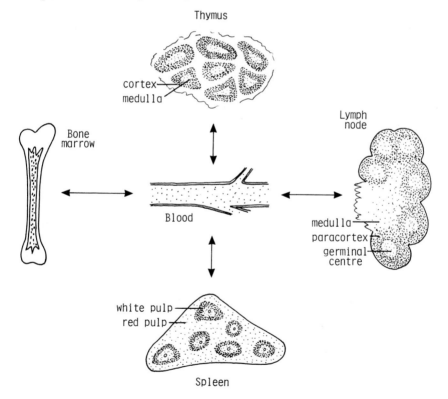

Figure 4.40. Anatomical organisation of the haemopoietic and lymphopoietic components of the haemolymphoreticular system.

and haemorrhagic lesions of the reproductive tract. Neoplasia may also increase the haemopoietic activity of the spleen, and mammary carcinomas often produce a striking response. Haemopoiesis therefore has many causes and is another example of one of the pitfalls that a toxicologist should be aware of when reviewing incidence summary data for evidence of treatment-related effects. Haemopoiesis usually appears as a single numerical entry, but each case may be related to entirely different causal circumstances, and low incidence, treatment-related cases may be masked when data from all causes are pooled for summary incidence tables. Finally, severe cases of haemopoiesis may be confused with neoplasia by pathologists unfamiliar with the mouse. Myelopoiesis can be extreme in some circumstances, and as well as obliterating the normal architecture of the spleen, large areas of proliferating myeloid cells may be found in lymph nodes and liver. These severe cases mimic granulocytic leukaemia and are often referred to as a 'leukaemoid response'.

Lymphoid hyperplasia, like haemopoiesis, is a common response to a wide variety of causes. The two main causes are inflammations and infections, particularly viral. In younger mice, the response to such insults is clear cut. The lymph nodes are enlarged, germinal centres are prominent and the medullary cords are packed with plasma cells. The architecture of the node may be distorted, but is still distinct, and there is little difficulty in distinguishing these acute reactive hyperplasias from neoplastic proliferations. In older mice, however, certain elements of the lymph node and splenic white pulp may proliferate in the absence of any obvious causal circumstances. These proliferations often resemble large distorted bizarre germinal centres; and such low grade chronic, possibly preneoplastic, hyperplasias in ageing mice are a further reflection of the disturbed immune system that forms the basis of much of the important pathology of this species.

Thymic hyperplasia can also be considered in the same general syndrome of chronic lymphoid proliferation of the ageing mouse. The thymus normally regresses in the first few months of life, but in ageing mice, particularly females, the medulla of one or both lobes often develops into a progressively proliferating lymph node-like structure with prominent germinal centres. The thymus may be enlarged at necropsy, and well-differentiated small lymphocytes are seen spilling into the surrounding tissues in sections examined histologically. The classification of these larger proliferations as hyperplasia or neoplasia is equivocal, but it is a distinctly different entity from the massive lethal blast cell proliferation of the younger mice described in the next section.

Neoplasia

Tumours of the haemolymphoreticular system, liver and lung account for about 80% of tumours in CD-1 mice. Blood vessel tumours and various tumours of the uterus account for a significant proportion of the remainder. Other tumour types rarely exceed 10% of tumour-bearing animals and, in contrast to rats, endocrine tumours are uncommon.

Haemolymphoreticular tumours

These are the most significant group of neoplasms both in terms of clinical symptoms and incidence and not least of all because of the diagnostic problems they create for the pathologist. A variety of classification schemes has been devised based on anatomy, cytology, cell-surface markers and various other parameters and each scheme has numerous proponents and antagonists. The sheer number of schemes in itself suggests that there is no ideal system and the validity of any scheme is simply its practical utility in the situation for which it is being used. In the context of regulatory toxicology the pathologist is presented with HE-stained samples from both scheduled and unscheduled sacrifices and is only required to establish whether the pattern of haemolymphoreticular neoplasia is affected by treatment. For this purpose, a simple analysis of the overall incidence of tumours and the major subgroups is all that is required. Further subdivisions and analyses are important in the further understanding of this area of neoplasia, but are of little significance in establishing treatment-related effects.

The older classification schemes were based primarily on the lineage of the proliferating cell together with the major site of the proliferation. This is a robust and reasonably practical classification in the context of toxicological pathology and can be easily subdivided by other parameters if minor patterns are of interest. The two primary sites of proliferation are in haemopoietic tissue (bone marrow and splenic red pulp) and lymphoid tissue (thymus, lymph node and splenic white pulp). The two basic diagnoses related to these sites are leukaemia (or leukosis) and lymphoma, respectively. The main proliferating cells encountered are the myeloid series in haemopoietic tissue and the lymphoid and histiocyte series in the solid lymphoid organs. A fairly simple classification scheme can be constructed on this basis to account for many of the haemolymphoreticular tumours of mice (Table 4.13).

Table 4.13. Common haemolymphoreticular tumours in mice.

Site	Cells	Diagnosis
Haemopoietic tissue	Undifferentiated	Leukaemia—undifferentiated
	Granulocytes	Leukaemia—granulocytic
Lymphoid tissue	Undifferentiated	Lymphoma—undifferentiated
	Lymphoid	Lymphoma—lymphocytic
	Histiocyte	Lymphoma—histiocytic
	Pleocellular	Lymphoma—mixed

This basic site and cell-type classification may be subdivided to provide more detailed patterns if required. For example, the lymphoid tissue site may be qualified as thymus or Peyer's patch, and the lymphoid cell series may be subdivided into plasmacytoid, immunoblastic or well-differentiated small lymphocyte. Unfortunately, such subdivisions are more than offset by a relatively large proportion of tumours of uncertain origin and lineage. Uncertainty of origin relates mainly to the widely disseminated undifferentiated cell which kills a significant proportion of mice in the first year. Some of these may be thymic and others haemopoietic in origin, but the usual picture is of total replacement of the haemolymphorecticular system by a uniform population of large, rapidly-dividing undifferentiated cells. Such a lack of differentiation also hinders any attempt at classifying neoplasia by cell of origin. Another confounding factor is autolysis. The rate of autolysis in mice is relatively rapid in comparison with the rat, and during autolysis nuclei either round up or fragment which may prevent the identification of proliferating cell lines. Despite these difficulties, the majority of cases can be diagnosed with reasonable certainty. The cytology of the classic forms is shown in Figure 4.41.

Granulocytic leukaemia (granulocytic leukosis) occurs in all age groups, but

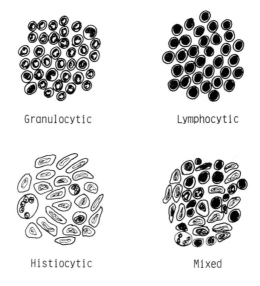

Granulocytic   Lymphocytic

Histiocytic   Mixed

Figure 4.41. Cytology of mouse haemolymphoreticular tumours.

is less frequent than the lymphoid tumours. Differentiation towards mature granulocytes tends to be more advanced in older mice and many cases can be diagnosed at necropsy by the green colour the proliferating cells impart to infiltrated lymph nodes (chloroleukaemia).

Tumours of the lymphoid series are the predominant tumours but they are a very diverse group with cell types ranging from undifferentiated blast cells to various mature forms such as small lymphocytes or plasma cells.

Histiocytic lymphomas (reticulum cell sarcoma type A) are a fairly distinct group except in their less-differentiated forms. They usually arise in the mesenteric lymph node or spleen, and infiltrates in the liver tend to form solid nests rather than the diffuse zonal infiltrations of other tumours. Other identifying features are a tendency to form pale acidophilic spindle cells in contrast to the round basophilic cell of lymphomas. Hyaline droplets in the renal proximal tubular epithelium are a frequent accompaniment of this tumour class. The MPS is widespread and the main problem with histiocytic tumours is a suitable terminology to include those arising in extralymphatic sites such as the liver, skin and uterus. The diagnosis histiocytic sarcoma is often used to indicate tumours arising from sites outside the solid lymphoid organs.

The final group of tumours arising in the solid lymphoid organs is the mixed lymphoma (composite lymphoma, reticulum cell sarcoma type B). This tumour often arises in the mesenteric lymph node and all types of haemolymphoreticular cells appear to be present including plasma cells, small lymphocytes, eosinophils, histiocytes and giant cells. The latter are probably the main diagnostic marker for this tumour, and some cases may resemble Hodgkin's disease in man. There is no consensus on which particular cell line is the neoplastic element and this is reflected in the use of the terms mixed or composite for this tumour.

Liver tumours (Figure 4.42)

Whilst haemolymphoreticular tumours are both interesting and controversial diagnostic challenges, they are less of a problem in regulatory toxicology than the mouse liver tumour. The financial impact of regulatory decisions based on treatment-related increases in the incidence of this one entity must be several billions of dollars and the controversy has yet to be resolved. The diagnostic terms used to describe these hepatocellular proliferations range from hyperplastic nodule to carcinoma, but most current literature favours a neoplastic rather than a hyperplastic status. However, the criteria used to differentiate benign from malignant tumours vary widely between pathologists and the ratio of benign to malignant tumours that appears on incidence summary tables can only be considered as an approximation. For this reason, some pathologists prefer a catch-all term such as hepatoma. This is consistent with the common practice of pooling certain categories of data for statistical analysis regardless of diagnosis.

Despite these uncertainties, pathologists can recognise different morphological patterns within this general class of hepatocellular proliferations and this is reflected in various classification schemes. These usually subdivide liver tumours into 2–4 classes on the basis of cytology, architecture, size and metastasis. Since metastasis is infrequent in most mouse strains, the first three parameters usually form the basis of most classification schemes. Small tumours (<5 mm) tend to be composed of basophilic hepatocytes forming a solid nodule or arranged as single-celled trabeculae, and they rarely metastasise. The cytoplasm is often vacuolated and may contain eosinophilic inclusions. This is generally considered the benign end of the spectrum, and terms used to describe it are Type 1, Type A, Grade 1 or adenoma. The larger tumours are often composed of plump hepatocytes, with abundant homogeneous cytoplasm, arranged in either solid nodules or in prominent multilayered trabeculae sometimes forming pseudoglandular

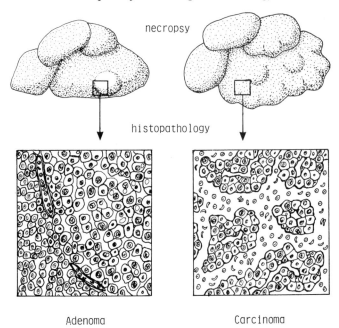

Figure 4.42. Mouse liver tumours.

patterns. Mitotic figures are usually more frequent than in smaller tumours, and it is the large tumour with plump hepatocytes arranged in prominent trabecular formations that tends to metastasise most frequently. This end of the spectrum is usually accepted as carcinoma. However, there is a considerable range between the microscopic tumour and the metastasising mass and defining class boundaries across the spectrum is somewhat subjective. The only point of definite agreement is that liver tumours are usually more frequent in males than in females. The significance of treatment-related increases in this common tumour of the mouse remains controversial.

Lung tumours

The classification of mouse lung tumours is subject to about the same degree of uncertainty as the diagnosis of liver tumours. Lung tumours occur with approximately equal frequency in both sexes and multiple tumours are common. The morphological spectrum ranges from microscopic or small subpleural nodules of round eosinophilic cells with few mitoses to large masses of plump basophilic cells arranged in papillary patterns (Figure 4.43). The latter often have foci of high mitotic rate, cause fibroplasia in the overlying pleura and may invade the mediastinum. The small eosinophilic nodule and rapidly dividing basophilic papillary mass may reasonably be diagnosed as adenoma and carcinoma respectively, but many tumours have an intermediate morphology, and class boundaries are difficult to define. For this reason, some pathologists consider all tumours

as carcinomas. Other pathologists use all-inclusive terms such as alveolar–bronchiolar neoplasm and subspecify tumours by the degree of differentiation or by
other qualifying terms. This is consistent with the tendency for some statisticians
and regulatory agencies to pool the data for analysis and review.

Other tumours

As in the rat, a diverse range of other types of epithelial and mesenchymal tumour
occurs, but the incidence of any one type rarely exceeds 10%. For data-handling
purposes they are considered as low frequency tumours. Blood-vessel tumours
present an interesting diagnostic and analytical dilemma. Vascular proliferations
are relatively common in mice, particularly in the liver, spleen and female reproductive tract. They often appear as dilated or cavernous vascular channels and present the common diagnostic problem of differentiating hyperplasia from neoplasia.
This difficulty is further complicated by the problem of grouping the tumours

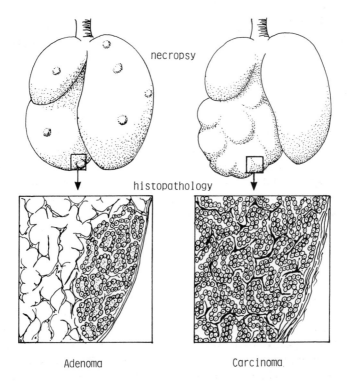

Figure 4.43. Mouse lung tumours.

for analysis. If haemangiomas are classified by the organs in which they occur,
then the incidence in any one organ is usually quite low. However, if they are considered to be tumours of blood vessels regardless of the organ in which they occur,

the incidence of haemangiomas may greatly increase. This problem is not unique to blood vessels and theoretically could apply to any mesenchymal element, but it illustrates once again the profound effect that classification systems can have on the way in which incidence data are presented. Thus, in the case of proliferative vascular lesions the incidence of neoplasia could range from zero, if the lesion is considered a non-neoplastic proliferation such as angiomatosis, to a high-frequency tumour if it is classified under the cardiovascular system as haemangioma.

Summary

The pathology of the ageing CD-1 mouse is similar to that of the Sprague-Dawley rat in that relatively few lesions are of major biological significance. Group housing and fighting is of major importance in males, and in females many lesions are related to the immune system in the form of amyloidosis, glomerulonephropathy and lymphoreticular neoplasia. Much of this is probably associated with viral infection of the lymphoreticular system and the manifestation of such infections will vary from strain to strain. In some strains, amyloidosis is virtually unknown, and in others immune-complex glomerulonephropathy is a major killer in early life. Similarly, some strains have a high incidence of thymic tumours in early life and others tend to develop a more widely disseminated chronic lymphoproliferative disease in later life. Similar variability occurs in the incidence of liver and lung tumours, and it cannot be stressed too often that the pathology of any one species is influenced so much by environment and genotype that the 'standard mouse' is extinct as far as the toxicologist is concerned. However, this should not deter a toxicologist from trying to define the major entities that dominate the background pathology of the strain that he is using. An understanding of this background is an important first step in assessing the significance of treatment-related effects.

Bibliography

General

Bartosek, I., Guaitani, A. and Pacei, E. (1982) *Animals in Toxicological Research*. (New York: Raven Press)

Benirschke, K., Garner, F. M. and Jones, T. C. (eds.) (1978) *Pathology of Laboratory Animals*, Vol. 1 and 2. (New York: Springer-Verlag)

Heywood, R. and Buist, D. P. (1983) The effects of health and health monitoring on toxicology studies. In *The Importance of Laboratory Animal Genetics, Health and the Environment in Biomedical Research*, edited by E. C. Melby and M. W. Balk (New York: Academic Press)

Ribelin, W. E. and McCoy, J. R. (1965) *Pathology of Laboratory Animals*. (Springfield: C. C. Thomas)

Rat and mouse

Anver, M. R., Cohen, B. J., Lattuada, C. P. and Foster, S. J. (1982) Age-associated lesions in barrier-reared male Sprague-Dawley rats: a comparison between HAP:(SD) and Crl:COBS(R) CD(R) SD stocks. *Exp. Aging Res.*, 8: 1.

Baker, H. J., Lindsey, J. R. and Weisbroth, S. H. (eds.) (1979) *The Laboratory Rat.* Vol. 1. *Biology and Diseases.* (New York: Academic Press).

Burek, J. D. (1978) *Pathology of Aging Rats.* (West Palm Beach: CRC Press)

Burek, J. D., Van der Kogel, A. J. and Hollander, C. F. (1976) Degenerative myelopathy in three strains of aging rats. *Vet. Pathol.*, 13: 321.

Butler, W. H. and Newberne, P. M. (eds.) (1975) *Mouse Hepatic Neoplasia.* (Amsterdam: Elsevier-North Holland).

Castleman, W. L. (1983) Respiratory tract lesions in weanling outbred rats infected with Sendai virus. *Am. J. Vet. Res.*, 44: 1024.

Cohen, B. J. and Anver, M. R. (1976) Pathological changes during aging in the rat. In *Special Review of Experimental Aging Research: Progress in Biology*, edited by M. F. Elias, B. E. Eleftheriou and P. K. Elias (Mt. Desert: Beech Hill)

Conner, M. W., Conner, B. H., Fox, J. G. and Rogers, A. E. (1983) Spontaneous amyloidosis in outbred CD-1 mice. *Survey Synth. Pathol. Res.*, 1: 67.

Cotchin, E. and Roe, F. J. C. (eds.) (1967) *Pathology of Laboratory Rats and Mice.* (Oxford: Blackwell)

Fong, A. C. O., Hardman, J. M. and Porta, E..A. (1982) Immunocytochemical hormonal features of pituitary adenomas of aging Wistar male rats. *Mech. Aging Develop. Res.*, 20: 141.

Foster, H. L., Fox, J., and Small, J. D. (eds.) (1982) *The Mouse in Biomedical Research.* Vol. 2. *Diseases.* (New York: Academic Press)

Frith, C. H., Highman, B., Burger, G. and Sheldon, W. D. (1983) Spontaneous lesions in virgin and retired breeder BALB/c and C57 BL/6 mice. *Lab. Anim. Sci.*, 33: 273.

Frith, C. H. and Ward, J. M. (1979) A morphologic classification of proliferative and neoplastic hepatic lesions in mice. *J. Environ. Pathol. Toxicol.*, 3: 329.

Frith, C. H. and Wiley, L. D. (1981) Morphologic classification and correlation of incidence of hyperplastic and neoplastic hematopoietic lesions in mice with age. *J. Gerontol.*, 36: 534.

Goodman, D. G., Ward, J. M., Squire, R. A., Chu, K. and Linhard, M. S. (1978) Neoplastic and non-neoplastic lesions in ageing F344 rats. *Toxicol. Appl. Pharmacol.*, 48: 237.

Gray, J. E. (1977) Chronic progressive nephrosis in the albino rat. *CRC Crit. Rev. Toxicol.*, 5: 115.

Gray, J. E., Van Zwieten, M. J. and Hollander, C. F. (1982). Early light microscopic changes of chronic progressive nephrosis in several strains of aging laboratory rats. *J. Gerontol.*, 37 142.

Greaves, P. and Faccini, J. M. (1984) *Rat Histopathology. A Glossary for use in Toxicity and Carcinogenicity Studies.* (Amsterdam: Elsevier Scientific)

Hackbarth, H. and Harrison, D. E. (1982) Changes with age in renal function and morphology in C57BL/6, CBA/HT6 and B6CBAF$_1$ mice. *J. Gerontol.*, 37: 540.

Heath, J. E., Frith, C. H. and Wang, P. M. M. (1982) A morphologic classification and incidence of alveolar-bronchiolar neoplasms in BALB/c female mice. *Lab. Anim. Sci.*, 32: 638.

International Expert Advisory Committee to the Nutrition Foundation (1983) *The Relevance of Mouse Liver Hepatoma to Human Carcinogenic Risk.* (Washington: Nutrition Foundation).

Kawada, K. and Ojima, A. (1978) Various epithelial and non-epithelial tumors spontaneously occurring in long-lived mice of A/St, CBA, C57BL/6 and their hybrid mice. *Acta Pathol. Jap.*, 28: 25.

Kolaja, G. J. and Fast, P.E. (1982) Renal lesions in MRL mice. *Vet. Pathol.*, 19: 663.

Komitowski, D., Sass, B. and Laub, W. (1982) Rat mammary tumor classification: notes on comparative aspects. *J. Nat. Cancer Inst.*, 68: 147.

Lohrke, H., Hesse, B. and Goerttler, K. (1982) Spontaneous tumours in male and female specified pathogen-free Sprague-Dawley (outbred stock SUT:SDT). *Z. Versuchstierkunde*, 24: 225.

Masoro, F. J. (1980) Mortality and growth characteristics of rat strains commonly used in aging research. *Exp. Aging Res.*, 6: 219.

Newberne, P. M. and Butler, W. H. (eds.) (1978) *Rat Hepatic Neoplasia.* (Cambridge: MIT Press)

Reuber, M. D., Vlahakis, G. and Heston, W. E. (1981) Spontaneous hyperplastic and neoplastic lesions of the uterus in mice. *J. Gerontol.*, 36: 661.

Sher, S. P. (1974) Tumors in control mice: literature tabulation. *Toxicol. Appl. Pharmacol.*, 30: 337.

Sher, S. P. Jensen, R. D. and Bokelman, D. L. (1982). Spontaneous tumours in control F344 and Charles River-CD rats and Charles River CD-1 and B6C3HF₁ mice. *Toxicol. Letts.*, 11: 103.

Solleveld, H. A., Haseman, J. K. and McConnell, E. E. (1984) Natural history of body weight gain, survival and neoplasia in the F344 rat. *J. Nat. Cancer Inst.*, 72: 929.

Suzuki, H., Mohr, U. and Kimmerle, G. (1979) Spontaneous endocrine tumors in Sprague-Dawley rats. *J. Cancer Res. Clin-Oncol.*, 95: 187.

Tarone, R. E., Chu, K. C. and Ward, J. M. (1981) Variability in the rates of some common naturally occurring tumors in Fischer F344 rats and (C57Bl/6N X C3H/HeN)Fᵢ (B6C3F) mice. *J. Nat. Cancer Inst.*, 66: 1175.

Turusov, V. S. (ed.) (1973) *Pathology of Tumours in Laboratory Animals*, Vol. 1/1. *Tumours of the Rat.* IARC Scientific Publication No. 5. (Lyon: International Agency for Cancer Research)

Turusov, V. S. (ed.) (1976) *Pathology of Tumours in Laboratory Animals*, Vol. 1/2. *Tumours of the Rat.* IARC Scientific Publication No. 6. (Lyon: International Agency for Cancer Research)

Turusov, V. S. (ed.) (1979) *Pathology of Tumours in Laboratory Animals*, Vol. 2. *Tumours of the Mouse.* IARC Scientific Publication, No. 23. (Lyon: International Agency for Research on Cancer)

Ward, J. M. (1983) Background data and variations in tumor rates of control rats and mice. *Prog. Exp. Tumor Res.*, 26: 241.

Ward, J. M., Goodman, D. G., Squire, R. A., Chu, K. C. and Linhard, M. S. (1979) Neoplastic and Non-neoplastic lesions in aging (C57BL/6N X C3H/HeN) F₁ (B6C3F₁) mice. *J. Nat. Cancer Inst.*, 63: 849.

Ward, J. M., Hamlin, M. H., Ackerman, L. J., Lattuada, C. P., Longfellow, D. G. and Cameron, T. P. (1983) Age related neoplastic and degenerative lesions in aging male virgin and ex-breeder ACl/segHapBR rats. *J. Gerontol.*, 38: 538.

Ward, J. M. and Vlahakis, G. (1978) Evaluation of hepatocellular neoplasms in mice. *J. Nat. Cancer Inst.*, 61: 807.

Yu, B. P., Masoro, E. J., Murata, I., Bertrand, H. A. and Lynd, F. T. (1982) Lifespan study of SPF Fischer-344 male rats fed *ad-libitum* or restricted diets — longevity, growth, lean body mass and disease. *J. Gerontol.*, 37: 130.

Other species

Abbott, D. P. and Majeed, S. K. (1984) A survey of parasitic lesions in wild-caught, laboratory-maintained primates: (Rhesus, Cynomolgus and Baboons). *Vet. Pathol.*, 21: 198.

Anderson, A. C. and Good, L. S. (eds.) (1970) *The Beagle as an Experimental Dog.* (Ames: Iowa University Press).

Bourne, G. H. (ed.) (1971) *The Rhesus Monkey*, Vol. 2. (New York: Academic Press)

Bourne, G. H. (1973) *Nonhuman Primates and Medical Research*. (New York: Academic Press)

Fiennes, R. N. T-W. (ed.) (1972) *Pathology of Simian Primates*. (Basel: Karger)

Graham, G. L. (1960) Parasitism in monkeys. *Ann. N.Y. Acad. Sci.*, 85: 842.

Homburger, F. (ed.) (1979) *The Syrian Hamster in Toxicology and Carcinogenesis Research*. (Basel: Karger)

Kuntz, R. E., Myers, B. J. and Moore, J. A. (1973) The baboon: parasitology. *Primates Med.*, 8: 79.

Lapin, B. A. and Yakovleva, L. A. (1963) *Comparative Pathology in Monkeys*. (Springfield: C. C. Thomas)

Mason, M. M. (1959) *Bibliography of the Dog*. (Ames: Iowa State University Press)

Mazue, G. and Richez, P. (1982) Problems in utilising monkeys in toxicology. In *Animals in Toxicological Research*, edited by I. Bartosek, A. Guaitani and E. Pacei (New York: Raven Press)

Pour, P., Althoff, J., Salmasi, S. Z. and Stepan, K. (1979) Spontaneous tumors and common diseases in three types of hamsters. *J. Nat. Cancer Inst.*, 63: 797.

Ruch, T. C. (1959) *Diseases of Laboratory Primates*. (Philadelphia: Saunders)

Schmidt, R. E. Eason, R. L., Hubbard, G. B., Young, J. T. and Eisenbrandt, D. L. (1983) *Pathology of Aging Syrian Hamsters*. (Boca Raton: CRC Press)

Toft, J. D. (1982) The pathophysiology of the alimentary tract and pancreas of nonhuman primates: a review. *Vet. Pathol.*, 19 (Suppl. 7): 44.

Vickers, J. H. (1969) Diseases of primates affecting the choice of species for toxicologic studies. *Ann. N.Y. Acad. Sci.*, 162: 659.

Wagner, J. E. and Manning, P. J. (eds.) (1976) *The Biology of the Guinea Pig*. (New York: Academic Press)

Weisbroth, S. H., Flatt, R. E. and Kraus, A. L. (eds.) (1974) *The Biology of the Laboratory Rabbit*. (New York: Academic Press)

5. Biostatistics in pathology

The problem posed to the toxicological pathologist in most situations is quite simple — what is the cause of the effect observed? The answer is usually arrived at through biological judgement based on experience, supported by statistical analysis. Many pathologists would place most emphasis on biological judgement, whereas non-pathologists are often more comfortable with statistically analysed data. Because of the importance of statistical techniques in analysing the relationships between cause and effect, some of the more common methods are briefly reviewed. The review refers mainly to regulatory toxicity studies in laboratory animals.

Statistical techniques have two main and interrelated applications in toxicology, experimental design and data analysis. In regulatory toxicology many important aspects of experimental design are more or less standardised in the form of guidelines issued by the regulatory agencies. These parameters include species, number of experimental groups, number of animals in each group, the range of dose levels to be used and the types of parameters to be assayed. Presently, the application of statistical techniques in experimental design is largely restricted to subsidiary applications for increasing precision and reducing error such as randomisation techniques and the construction of certain block designs.

In pathology, the main statistical considerations in experimental design are consistency in sampling tissues and consistency in observing and recording abnormalities in these tissues. Consistency in sampling means removing the same number of samples from the same organ sites for histological processing and examination. In some organs such as the lung or liver, lesions may not be distributed uniformly across all lobes and bias, or even missing lesions completely, can only be avoided by consistent sampling procedures. There are two aspects to reporting consistently. The first is to ensure that all lesions detected at necropsy are commented upon histopathologically. The second is to avoid observer drift. There are several ways of avoiding drift. One is to examine slides 'blind', i.e. without knowledge of the treatment the animals received. Many pathologists consider this leads to insensitivity in their observation, and it is more usually done in re-evaluations than as a first step. Other pathologists examine slides using statistical designs such as replicate blocking or random sequences. Increasing in vogue, with the advent of computers, is the use of prompts. As each organ is examined the pathologist is presented with a list of standard common lesions from which to select his diagnosis. Many pathologists still rely on 'self-discipline', but this may weaken during the evaluation of large numbers of tissues or be destroyed by numerous interruptions during the working day. The majority of statistical input, however, is on the data at the end of the experiment, using well-defined analytical methods.

Analytical methods

The two main types of data generated in regulatory toxicity studies are quantitative data and quantal data. Quantitative data are sometimes referred to as continuous or semi-continuous data. They are the sort of data generated in clinical chemistry or haematology where every animal or assay produces a result. Organ weights are another example of quantitative data; for example, every animal has a liver and every liver has a weight. Analysis of organ weights and similar data is frequently based on a comparison of the location and scatter of data between control and treated groups. Commonly used tests include Student's *t*-test, analysis of variance, Wilcoxon's sum of ranks test and the Kruskal–Wallis test. Details of these tests for quantitative data can be found in standard statistical texts and are not considered further.

With the main exception of organ weights, most data in pathology are quantal. These data are sometimes referred to as discrete data or dichotomous data. The animal may or may not have the effect of interest such as a particular type of neoplasm. Within any group of animals the data can be expressed either as an incidence of affected animals e.g. 5 out of 10, or as a proportion of affected animals e.g. 0.5 or 50%. Statistical analysis of quantal data are often based on the comparison of the proportion of affected animals in control and treated groups. In short-term toxicity studies, animals are usually killed at scheduled times and Chi-squared (χ^2) and Fisher's exact test are commonly used to analyse the data. In long-term carcinogenicity studies, animals often die or are removed because of illness before study termination, and some adjustment is required to allow for variable survival. The Fisher's exact test is difficult to adjust for mortality and variants of the Chi-squared test are used. The log-rank test is one variant, but another variant, the test for positive trend, is becoming increasingly used.

Chi-squared (χ^2)

This is a simple test based on the principle of comparing observed (O) with expected (E) frequencies. The bigger the difference in proportions between control and treated groups, the less likely is the difference to be due to chance. For example, it is very likely that finding 5 out of 10 affected rats in both treated and control groups is due to chance; whereas, it is unlikely to be a chance effect if 9 out of 10 treated rats have a lesion compared with 1 out of 10 controls. The method of calculating the χ^2 statistic can be found in most statistical texts and will not be detailed here. It is based essentially on the ratio $(O-E)^2/E$. Chi-squared is only valid for the more frequent lesions and the expected number should be at least five cases in each group. For smaller frequencies the test has to be adjusted using Yates' correction, or Fisher's exact test should be used.

Fisher's exact test

This test is used when the number of lesions is too small for a Chi-squared test. It is used in what is termed a four-fold table or 2×2 contingency table. This table compares two groups, and within each group presents the number of animals with and without the lesion of interest (Table 5.1).

Fisher's test is based on the discovery that the exact probability of getting any particular values by chance in such a table can be calculated by using a certain hypergeometric formula. The greater the difference between the two groups in the incidence of lesions, the less likely is this to be due to chance and Fisher's test is used to calculate such probabilities.

Table 5.1.　Incidence of a lesion in two groups of 10 animals presented as a four-fold table.

	Control group	Treated group	Total
Lesion present	2	7	9
Lesion absent	8	3	11
Total	10	10	20

Test for positive trend

This test is one recommended by the International Agency for Cancer Research for analysing data from long-term carcinogenicity studies. Like the Chi-squared test, it is based on the comparison of observed and expected frequencies of lesions, but it incorporates three important modifications. It takes account of animals dying during the study. This is important for the simple reason that tumour development is a long process and animals killed early in the study are less likely to have tumours than those killed at the end. Thus, if treated animals tend to die earlier than controls because of toxicity, then simply adding up the number of animals with tumours may lead to a statistically significant increase in tumour incidence in controls because the treated animals did not live long enough to develop any tumours. Secondly, it uses the data from all dose groups to assess for dose-related trends in frequencies, hence the name 'positive trend' (with respect to dose). Finally, it incorporates a modification to adjust the analysis for lesions that are fatal and those that are non-fatal such as minor or incidental lesions. Lethal tumours are analysed by the so-called 'death rate' method and incidentally observed tumours by the 'prevalence' method. These analyses are used to derive the P-value for positive trend with respect to dose. The latter modification is somewhat controversial in that it requires the pathologist to categorise lesions as fatal or non-fatal. This is often less difficult than it may appear and as described in Chapter 4 the cause of illness of about 90% of rodents could be assigned with reasonable certainty. In any case, the analysis does allow for uncertainty in the use of the categories 'probably fatal' and 'probably non-fatal', or simply a single category 'uncertain'.

Analytical problems

Statistical analyses of experimental data may be very powerful tools, but their application in toxicological pathology has certain problems. The main problems are classification of data, sample size and the fundamental nature of cause–effect relationships.

Data classification

Statistical techniques are precise mathematical methods, but the data to which they are applied are often far from precise. Statistical tests are applied to discrete numbers. Diagnostic terms on the other hand usually reflect categorisation within a spectrum or range of dynamic responses. There may be some uncertainty or variability in the diagnostic criteria used to set class boundaries within this range. Several examples of uncertainty were described in Chapter 4, particularly with respect to proliferations. An extreme example of classification problems in carcinogenicity studies would be the classification of some proliferative lesions as hyperplasias rather than neoplasias. This may be reasonable in some tissues, but it means that the data for the organ could be zero and not analysed if one sticks rigidly to analysis of tumour data only. A more subtle problem is the effect of categorisation within a range. Mouse liver tumours range from microscopic nodules to gross metastasising masses. These are frequently classified into two or more discrete classes, such as benign and malignant tumours. Such splitting may produce low-incidence categories which in themselves may be too small to analyse for statistically significant differences. On the other hand, the pooling of all data into one category 'liver proliferations' may reveal highly significant differences. This ability to alter statistical significance by changing the classification system is of course highly controversial. It is not surprising therefore that regulatory agencies tend to advise data pooling since this gives the most conservative view on which to base predictions of risk to man or other species.

Sample size

The number of animals used in regulatory toxicology is a major limitation in statistical analyses. Non-rodent studies generally have 3–5 animals/sex/group, and this clearly limits the power of statistical analyses. Short-term rodent studies are a little better, using 10–20 animals/sex/group, but this is not without its problems, and neither is the use of 50 animals/sex/group in long-term rodent studies. A crude significance test is presented in Table 5.2 which is a guideline to the magnitude of difference required between the incidences of lesions in control and treated groups to achieve statistical significance at $P<0.05$. It must be stressed that this table is only a crude guide to show the approximate statistical resolving power of different-sized experiments and it should not be used as a formal statistical test.

Table 5.2.   Number of lesions in treated group required to achieve statistical significance for different numbers of lesions in control groups ($P<0.05$).

Group size 10		Group size 20		Group size 50	
Control	Treated	Control	Treated	Control	Treated
0	5	0	6	0	6
1	7	1	7	1	7
2	8	2	9	5	13
3	9	4	11	10	19
4	10	8	15	20	30
5	10	12	18	30	40

Two important points should be evident from this table. The first is that increasing the group size from 10 to 50 per group does not have much effect on the differences required between incidence levels when dealing with uncommon lesions. For example, if there is one lesion in the control group you need about seven cases in the treated group for significance regardless of group size. The converse of this point is that a group size of 10 is relatively insensitive for detecting statistical significance when there are background lesions in controls. All the treated animals have to be affected for statistical significance if there are 3–5 cases in the controls and if there are more than five cases it is impossible to attain statistical significance. Statistics are therefore of limited utility in short-term toxicity studies in which group sizes of 10 or less are frequently used.

   The second point highlights a difference between biological interpretation and statistical interpretation. Statistical interpretation is based largely on the *difference* between numbers in the control and treated groups ($O-E$) whereas the biologist's thought processes are often based on *multiples* of the incidence in control values. For example, in tumour analysis in groups of 50 animals, with control incidences ranging from 5 to 30/group the difference between control and treated group is in the range 8–10 cases at all levels. However, the pathologist may view 5 *vs.* 13 as an increase of 160% whereas 20 *vs.* 30 is only a 50% increase. This is one reason for the dichotomy of opinion in analyses of tumour data. A doubling of the incidence of an uncommon tumour from 5 to 10 cases will not be statistically significant, but may appear highly significant to a pathologist. On the other hand, a pathologist may not feel too concerned about a 50% increase in the incidence of a common tumour such as rat mammary tumours, but this may be statistically significant. Biological significance may thus appear to be inversely correlated with statistical significance and resolution of this dichotomy may pose serious problems for regulatory agencies who have to act on the basis of such data.

Sample size also affects decision-making on the so-called 'no-effect level'. Most studies incorporate several dose levels in an attempt to establish a dose-response relationship. The no-effect level is usually based on the highest dose level in which no observable response is detected. The certainty that can be placed in this decision largely depends on the number of animals used at that dose level. This sample size determines the probability of both observing a response for a given incidence in the population and conversely the probability of missing a response when one really exists at this dose level. This can be termed the 'detection sensitivity' of the sample (Tables 5.3 and 5.4).

Table 5.3. Probability of a given sample of animals containing at least one affected case for different background incidence levels.

Sample size	'True' population incidence level (%)				
	2	5	10	20	40
10	0.183	0.402	0.652	0.893	0.994
20	0.333	0.642	0.879	0.989	1.0
30	0.455	0.786	0.958	0.999	1.0
50	0.636	0.923	0.995	1.0	1.0

Table 5.3 shows that by using a sample size of 10 there is only an 18% probability of detecting at least one event when the background population incidence is 2%, but over a 90% probability of observing at least one affected animal when 40% of the population have the lesion of interest.

For assessment of no-effect levels, the more important question is the probability that nil cases in a group is really a true zero. An approximate upper confidence limit for background incidence levels from which a nil case sample could be drawn is presented in Table 5.4. As an example, there is still a 1 in 20 chance of getting zero cases in a sample of 10 rats drawn from a population containing 26% affected animals. In other words, the result 0/10 in a group does not mean that the dose is a no-effect level, but that less than 26% of the animals in an infinitely sized experiment would be likely to show a response at that dose.

Current experimental designs using a control and three dose levels and samples of 50 or less animals/sex/group do not therefore allow statements of no-effect levels to be made with any degree of confidence. To make matters worse, the examples quoted above were based on the detection of discrete well-defined responses which did not occur in controls. In reality, many responses are not so well defined, and similar lesions may be present in controls. For example, spontaneous renal disease may confound the detection of low-grade toxic nephropathy

Table 5.4. Maximum background incidence that could yield a zero result in a sample ($P<0.05$).

Sample size (n)	5	10	15	20	50
Background incidence (%)	45	26	18	14	6

in older rats, and the increasing incidence of spontaneous tumours in ageing controls may make statistical evaluation of tumours in treated groups less sensitive as the experiment is extended from 18 months to a lifetime study. Increasing sample size is the obvious answer to these problems, but this would have to go into the hundreds or thousands to show any substantial effect on the sensitivity of current experimental designs. This would be impossible to justify both ethically and financially and toxicologists and statisticians will have to work within the restrictions imposed by small groups.

Causal associations

In many cases, statistically significant differences between control and treated groups are associated with treatment. However, the association between cause and effect may not always be straight forward. This final section of the book briefly reviews some of the factors that the pathologist has to consider when evaluating causal associations suggested by the results of statistical tests.

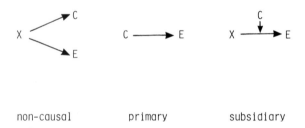

Figure 5.1. Simple patterns of causal association. C = Cause; E = Effect; X = Other factor.

In their simplest form statistical associations may be non-causal or causal. The latter may be primary or subsidiary (Figure 5.1). Non-causal associations are frequent in epidemiological studies of cause–effect relationships. They usually result from association of events being measured with a third unknown factor (Factor X). For example, an increase in heart disease (E) in a population may be statistically associated with an increase in a suspected causal factor (C) such as motor-car driving, but in reality both are associated with general affluence (factor X) and the association between C and E is non-causal. This problem, sometimes called the ecological fallacy, may also occur in toxicology. For example, hormone imbalance due to a large pituitary tumour may lead to testicular atrophy. The tumour may also compress the brain leading to inanition, stress and gastritis. The incidence of gastritis may correlate well with the incidence of testicular atrophy, but gastritis does not cause testicular atrophy or vice versa. They are related via pituitary tumours as a common causal factor. This common factor would not, however, be discovered if the cranial cavity was not examined at necropsy, and incorrect conclusions could be drawn from statistically correlated data.

Primary causal associations are more common in toxicology. If a large dose of cyanide causes death, this may seem to be a primary direct causal association. However, directness depends on the depth of our current state of knowledge. Cyanide disrupts electron transfer, which stops oxidative phosphorylation. This stops the heart and death ensues. In reality the pathologist has to consider a chain of causations, and it may be difficult to distinguish the primary from the secondary effects. For example, a chemical may chronically damage the kidney and secondary lesions may occur in the cardiovascular system. If atrial thrombosis occurs, the heart stops and death ensues. This is a slight variant of the cyanide example, but what is the causal relationship between the chemical and a statistically significant increase in the incidence of atrial thrombosis? In the above examples, the chain of causation is known, but in experimental work on novel chemicals, the pathologist may have difficulty deciding which step of the chain is being observed.

The same difficulty applies to the study of subsidiary causal effects. In these cases, the chemical modifies an underlying process. Several examples of this were described in the young rat in Chapter 4 such as chemical exacerbation of respiratory disease caused by *C. kutscheri*. A problem of more concern is in carcinogen bioassays. A treatment-related increase in the incidence of a common spontaneous tumour such as mouse liver tumours or rat mammary tumours is a frequent result. In many cases the chemical appears to have a subsidiary or modifying role in the process of carcinogenesis rather than act as a complete carcinogen. This is recognised in the increasing use of terms such as genotoxic and non-genotoxic carcinogens to differentiate between causal associations in data interpretation.

Although primary and subsidiary causal associations are valid concepts, the relationship between cause and effect may be extremely complex and involve both primary and subsidiary mechanisms. There may be several chains involved and several interacting or modifying factors in each chain. In fact, many effects are not dependent on single causes and it is often more appropriate to think in terms of an interwoven web of causation. If pathology, as is often stated, is an art rather than a science, the art lies in untangling the web of cause-effect relationships which are the foundation of toxicological pathology.

Bibliography

Fears, T. R. and Douglas, J. F. (1977) Suggested procedures for reducing the pathology workload in a carcinogen bioassay program. *Environ. Pathol. Toxicol.*, 1: 125.

Gad, S. C. and Weil, C. S. (1982) Statistics for toxicologists. In *Principles and Methods of Toxicology*, edited by W. A. Hayes (New York: Raven Press)

Gart, J. J., Chu, K. and Tarone, R. E. (1979) Statistical issues in interpretation of chronic bioassay tests for carcinogenicity. *J. Nat. Cancer Inst.*, 62: 957.

Hewlett, P. S. and Plackett, R. L. (1979) *The Interpretation of Quantal Responses in Biology* (Baltimore: University Park Press)

Kodell, R. L., Farmer, J. H., Gaylor, D. W. and Cameron, A. M. (1982) Influence of cause-of-death assignment on time-to-tumor analyses in animal carcinogenesis testing. *J. Nat. Cancer Inst.*, 69: 659.

Peto, R., Pike, M. C., Day, N. E., Gray, R. G., Lee, P. N., Parish, S., Peto, J., Richards, S. and Wahrendorf, J. (1980) Guidelines for simple, sensitive significance tests for carcinogenic effects in long-term animal experiments. In *Long-term and Short-term Screening Assays for Carcinogens: a Critical Appraisal*. International Agency for Research on Cancer (IARC) Monographs, suppl. 2, Annex. (Lyon: World Health Organisation).

Portier, C. and Hoel, D. (1983) Optimal design of the chronic animal bioassay. *J. Toxicol. Environ. Health*, 12: 1.

Roe, F. J. C. (1981) Testing *in vivo* for general chronic toxicity and carcinogenicity. In *Testing for Toxicity*, edited by J. W. Gorrod (London: Taylor and Francis)

Salsburg, D. S. (1979) Research design from the biostatisticians viewpoint. *Clin. Toxicol.*, 15: 559.

Ward, J. M. and Reznik, G. (1983) Refinements of rodent pathology and the pathologists' contribution to evaluation of carcinogenesis bioassays. *Prog. Exp. Tumor Res.*, 26: 266.

Weil, C. S. (1973) Experimental design and interpretation of data from prolonged toxicity studies. In *Pharmacology and the Future of Man*, edited by T. A. Loomis (Basel: Karger)

Weinburger, M. (1980) How valuable is blind evaluation in histopathologic examinations in conjunction with animal toxicity studies? *Toxicol. Pathol.*, 7: 14.

Index

213

Statistics, 204–212
  blind evaluation, 204
  causal associations, 210
  chi-squared, 205
  data classification, 207
  Fisher's exact test, 206
  sample sizes, 207
  test for postive trend, 206
Steatosis, 23
  see also specific organs
  hormones and, 86
  staining for, 24
Stomach
  see also GI tract
  Abbreviata sp. in, 156
  adaptive cytoprotection, 77
  adenomatous hyperplasia, 190
  diffuse gastritis, 78
  erosion, 77
  forestomach hyperplasia, 75
  fundic hyperplasia, 78
  haemorrhage, 77
  mineralisation in dog, 146
  mucosal prostaglandins, 76
  Nochtia sp. in, 157
  NSAI's and, 76
  ulcer, 78
Streptomycin, and protein synthesis, 10
  and serum sickness, 20
Stria vascularis, 115
Sulphonamides, serum sickness, 20, 121
  leucopenia, 124
  renal toxicity, 101
Sulphur dioxide, asthma, 66
  airway metaplasia, 65
Superoxide anion, 12
Superoxide dismutase, 12
Synaptopathy, 109
  and amine analogues, 109
  and excitotoxins, 109

Tapetal necrosis, 114
Telangiectasis
  in dog spleen, 147
  in heart valves, 147
  in rat adrenal, 170
  in rat liver, 170
Terminology, construction of, 44–47
Testis
  atrophy, 18, 169

in ageing mouse, 189
  in ageing rat, 169
  in young baboon, 153
  in young dog, 150
  in cynomolgus monkey, 154
  in young rat, 139
  methallibur, 18
Tetracycline, and lipid, 79, 85
Thallium, cataract, 113
Thrombosis, 16
Thyroid
  C-cell hyperplasia, 150
  C-cell tumours, 181
  ectopic thymus, 135, 146, 153
TOCP, axonopathy, 108
Toluene diisocyanate, 14, 65
Toxascaris leonina, 150
Toxocara canis, 150
Tracheitis, 65
Trematodes, 157
  schistosomiasis, 157
  Paragonimus sp., 158
  Watsonius sp., 158
Trend test, 206
Triglyceride cycle, 86
Tubulin, 10
Tumours
  see neoplasia

Ulcer
  see specific organs
Uterus
  cyclic distension, 140
  cystic endometrial hyperplasia, 190

Vacuolation,
  in cornea, 60
  fatty, *see* steatosis
Vapour, 63
Vasodilation, 37
Vinca alkaloids, 10
  and neuronopathy, 107
Virus infections
  parvovirus, 152
  SDA, 142
  Sendai, 142

Wallerian degeneration, 108
Watsonius sp., 158
Whipworms, 156